The
DASH
Diet
HEALTH PLAN

Low-Sodium, Low-Fat Recipes
to Promote Weight Loss,
Lower Blood Pressure,
and Help Prevent Diabetes

ROCKRIDGE PRESS

TABLE OF CONTENTS

Introduction   1

**Section One: What You Need to Know About
the DASH Diet?**   3

    Chapter 1: What is the DASH Diet?   5

    Chapter 2: An Overview of the DASH Diet Plan   10

Section Two: How the DASH Diet Works   13

    Chapter 3: The DASH Diet's Effect on Your Health   15

    Chapter 4: Is the DASH Diet Right for You?   21

Section Three: DASH to a Better Lifestyle   23

    Chapter 5: Planning Your DASH Diet   25

    Chapter 6: Transitioning to the DASH Diet   31

Section Four: Your DASH Diet Eating Plan   37

    Chapter 7: Calorie Requirements & Food Guide   39

    Chapter 8: The DASH Diet Foods & Shopping Guide   42

    Chapter 9: The DASH Diet Menu Plans   51

Section Five: DASH to Fitness   73

    Chapter 10: Your 28-Day DASH to Fitness
Workout Plan   75

Section Six: The DASH Diet Cookbook   **83**

    Chapter 11: Breakfast   85

    Chapter 12: Lunch   108

    Chapter 13: Snacks & Appetizers   133

    Chapter 14: Dinner   156

    Chapter 15: Dessert   178

Conclusion   **203**

Appendix   **205**

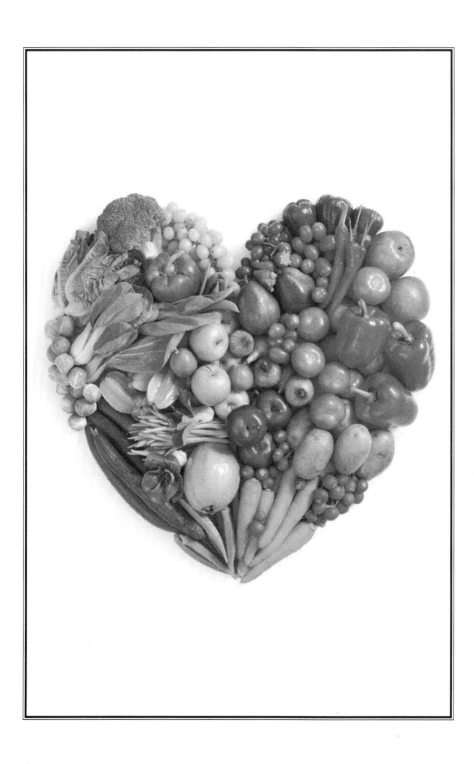

INTRODUCTION

I magine indulging in rosemary chicken, chocolate cake, berry banana smoothies, seafood fettuccine and French dip sandwiches. Now, imagine doing this while lowering your blood pressure, losing weight and reducing your risk of heart disease, stroke and diabetes. All of this—and more—is possible on the DASH diet.

Whether your goal is to eat healthy or to lose weight, the DASH diet is an excellent choice. It will help you get slim, fit and healthy with no gimmicks, hard to follow rules or restrictions. Instead of being stuck in the diet doldrums, you will feel satisfied and full of energy.

US News & World Report picked the DASH diet as its number one choice in Best Diets Overall, Best Diets for Healthy Eating and Best Diabetes Diets. It is nutritionally sound, based on extensive scientific research and has received widespread support and approval from the health community.

The DASH diet is not a fad diet or a crash diet. It's a medically developed plan that was designed to improve your health. On the DASH diet you can feel as good on the inside as you look on the outside.

The DASH diet is popular because it addresses health first and foremost. It has been shown to have a significant impact on hypertension (high blood pressure), cholesterol levels and even kidney function. Since the DASH diet is also an excellent weight loss plan, it has a beneficial impact on heart disease, type 2 diabetes, metabolic syndrome and other obesity-related conditions.

The DASH Diet Health Plan includes everything you need to succeed. We've streamlined the details to make the program as easy and enjoyable as possible. You'll find all the information you need, as well as meal plans, recipes and a quick-start fitness program. But it's not "one size fits all." In fact, you can customize the plan to meet your individual needs.

What You Need to Know About the DASH Diet

- **Chapter 1:** What is the DASH Diet?

- **Chapter 2:** An Overview of the DASH Diet Plan

WHAT IS THE DASH DIET?

The History of the DASH Diet

In response to the growing problem of high blood pressure in the US, the National Institutes of Health (NIH) provided funding in 1992 for research into a dietary solution to hypertension. The goal was to create Dietary Approaches to Stop Hypertension (DASH).

The National Heart, Lung and Blood Institute (NHLBI) conducted this research with the help of five of the most respected medical research institutions in the country:

- Johns Hopkins University
- Duke University Medical Center
- Kaiser Permanente Center for Health Research
- Brigham and Women's Hospital
- Pennington Biomedical Research Center

Together, these five facilities conducted the most extensive and exhaustive research to date on nutritional solutions for the growing problem of hypertension.

How the Studies Were Conducted

Teams of doctors, nutritionists, nurses and statisticians worked cooperatively between their respective institutions on randomized control trials. Each facility chose and studied its own groups of participants to ensure the most accurate research results. Over 8,000 people went through the screening process, and the researchers specifically sought to fill at least two-thirds of the spots with people at high risk of hypertension. At each facility, three diets were used to test the effect of a particular diet on blood pressure.

The first, or control diet, was a diet very close to the typical American diet: low in potassium, calcium, magnesium and fiber, with the same protein and fat intake of the average American diet. However, the control diet had a lower sodium intake (1500 mg) than the average diet, and its purpose was to represent the recommendation by doctors to lower sodium intake in order to lower blood pressure.

The second diet was similar to the control diet, but with more fruits and vegetables and fewer snacks. It was also higher in fiber.

The third diet, which became known as the DASH diet, was higher in fruits, vegetables, low-fat dairy and lean protein. It was also lower in saturated fat and overall fat intake. The DASH diet was based on research that showed that a high intake of fiber and certain minerals could have a very positive impact on high blood pressure.

The second and third diets included a daily sodium intake of 3,000 mg to represent the average sodium intake of Americans. The researchers wanted to see if nutritional changes other than lowering sodium intake could have a positive impact on hypertension.

Two DASH trials were conducted. The first ran from August 1993 to July 1997. The second, a DASH-Sodium trial, was conducted from September 1997 through November 1999.

During each of the two studies, each group was placed on the control diet for three weeks. Their blood pressure, urine and symptoms were monitored. At the end of this screening process, over 400 participants were chosen to continue in the study. Each participant was randomly assigned to one of the three diets for the duration of the study.

There was one difference between the first study and the second. The results of the first study showed that the control diet, with its low sodium intake, was effective in lowering blood pressure. The DASH diet was also effective, to a lesser degree. Thus, in the second research study, the DASH diet was redesigned to include the lower sodium intake, effectively combining the original DASH diet and the control diet. Because of this, the new DASH diet used in the second study was called the DASH-Sodium diet.

Conclusions

At the end of the second research study, the results showed that the control diet reduced blood pressure, but the new DASH-Sodium diet reduced it even more than the control diet or the original DASH diet. Researchers had found the right combination: the DASH diet (high fiber, low-fat dairy, plenty of fresh fruits and vegetables, lean protein) plus the lower sodium intake.

What the researchers discovered at all five research facilities was that this combination of the DASH diet and a reduced sodium intake of 1,500 mg/day resulted in an average blood pressure reduction of 8.9/4.5 mm Hg (systolic/diastolic) in people who were considered "pre-hypertensive." The hypertensive participants had an average reduction of 11.5/5.7 mm Hg. These results were after just 30 days on the DASH-Sodium diet.

These studies, along with additional research, showed that the DASH diet not only reduced blood pressure, but also reduced cholesterol and lowered body fat, particularly around the abdomen. This is due in part to the low sugar intake. (Reducing sugar in the diet improves insulin sensitivity. Once the body starts responding more to insulin, it will increasingly dispose of or use stored belly fat and the fat that you take in through your diet.)

These findings are the reason that the DASH diet is recommended by medical organizations such as the American Medical Association, the American Heart Association and many others.

Who Supports the DASH Diet and Why?

The DASH diet is endorsed by:

- The National Heart, Lung and Blood Institute[1]
- The American Heart Association (AHA)
- The 2010 Dietary Guidelines for Americans
- US Guidelines for Treatment of High Blood Pressure
- The 2011 AHA Treatment Guidelines for Women
- The Mayo Clinic[2, 3]

These agencies and medical institutions have recommended the DASH diet because of the many positive effects it can have on your health:

- Lowered intake of saturated fats and cholesterol is known to reduce the risk of both heart disease and arterial disease.
- Increased intake of healthy fats, such as Omega-3s, is known to increase heart health and also aid in the loss of fat around the abdomen, which reduces the risk of metabolic syndrome and type 2 diabetes.
- Lowering high blood pressure reduces the risk of heart attack and stroke.

"*Rigorous studies show DASH can lower blood pressure, which, if too high, can trigger heart disease, heart failure, and stroke. (In fact, the name DASH stands for Dietary Approaches to Stop Hypertension—hypertension being the medical term for high blood pressure.) It's also been shown to increase "good" HDL cholesterol and decrease "bad" LDL cholesterol and triglycerides, a fatty substance that in excess has been linked to heart disease. Overall, DASH reflects the medical community's widely accepted definition of a heart-healthy diet—it is heavy on fruits and vegetables and light on saturated fat, sugar, and salt.*"

– US News & World Report

The 2012 Dietary Guidelines for Americans recommend the DASH eating plan for everyone, including children and the elderly. The DASH diet even formed the basis for the MyPlate dietary guidelines (the new food pyramid) generated by the United States Department of Agriculture (USDA).

AN OVERVIEW OF THE DASH DIET PLAN

- **Reduces sodium to lower hypertension** or the risk of hypertension. Choose the standard DASH diet that allows up to 2300 milligrams (mg) of sodium per day or a low-sodium version that allows up to 1500 mg of sodium per day. The "typical" American diet includes as much as 3500 mg of sodium per day!
- **Increases fiber to reduce blood pressure,** steady blood sugar levels and aid in weight loss. The DASH diet provides more fresh fruits and vegetables than most people are used to eating, as well as a healthy selection of whole grains.
- **Reduces saturated fat and trans fat** in order to increase heart health, lower LDL (bad) cholesterol, raise HDL (good) cholesterol, aid in weight loss and decrease risks and symptoms of heart disease, diabetes and metabolic syndrome. Trans fats (from processed and fried foods) are omitted and foods low in saturated fats, such as low-fat dairy, lean meats and seafood are encouraged.
- **Increases healthy fats,** such as Omega-3s, by eating nuts, seeds, fish, avocado and other Omega-3 rich foods.
- **Helps reduce blood pressure** by limiting alcohol and caffeine.
- **Ensures proper levels of the minerals** shown to reduce high blood pressure, such as potassium and magnesium. Eating a wide variety

of foods containing minerals, such as bananas, legumes (beans) and leafy greens boosts mineral intake.

- **Reduces the risk of type 2 diabetes** and metabolic syndrome while lowering abdominal fat (a leading indicator of both). Sugary foods are limited to no more than five per week.

The DASH diet offers flexibility not just in sodium, but also in overall caloric intake.

You can choose menu plans that allow either 2300 mg or 1500 mg of sodium per day. People with high blood pressure or high risk of hypertension are advised to choose the lower intake of sodium.

The DASH Diet Health Plan serves a wide range of caloric needs:

Food Group	1,200 Calories	2,000 Calories	3,100 Calories
Grains[1]	4–5	6–8	12–13
Vegetables	3–4	4–5	6
Fruits	3–4	4–5	6
Fat free or low-fat dairy products[2]	2–3	2–3	3–4
Lean meats, poultry, and fish	3 or less	6 or less	6–9
Nuts, seeds, and legumes	3 per week	4–5 per week	1
Fats and oils[3]	1	2–3	4
Sweets and added sugars	3 or less per week	5 or less per week	≤2
Maximum sodium limit[4]	2,300 mg/day	2,300 mg/day	2,300 mg/day

Fig. 2.1. This table estimates the numbers of servings that you are allowed to have from each food group per day (unless noted otherwise). You can choose to follow a diet that is anywhere from 1600–3100 calories per day, depending on your calorie needs. Learn how to identify your calorie needs in Chapter 5.

(Table courtesy of the National Heart, Lung and Blood Institute of Health.)

[1] Whole grains are recommended for most grain servings as a good source of fiber and nutrients.

[2] For lactose intolerance, try either lactase enzyme pills with dairy products or lactose-free or lactose-reduced milk.

[3] Fat content changes the serving amount for fats and oils. For example, 1 Tablespoon regular salad dressing = one serving; 1 Tablespoon low-fat dressing = one-half serving; 1 Tablespoon fat-free dressing = zero servings.

[4] The DASH eating plan has a sodium limit of either 2,300 mg or 1,500 mg per day.

How the DASH Diet Works

- **Chapter 3:** The DASH Diet's Effect on Your Health

  - **Chapter 4:** Is the DASH Diet Right for You?

THE DASH DIET'S EFFECT ON YOUR HEALTH

U nlike most diet plans, the DASH diet wasn't created as a means of losing weight; it was designed to reduce high blood pressure, which in turn helps prevent heart disease and stroke.

Let's take a more in-depth look at how following the DASH diet can significantly improve your health.

The DASH Diet and High Blood Pressure

Following the DASH diet plan—particularly the low sodium version of the diet—has been shown to have a direct impact on high blood pressure. This combination of specific nutrients with a low sodium intake has produced significant positive results in every major study conducted.

"By following the DASH diet, you may be able to reduce your blood pressure by a few points in just two weeks. Over time, your blood pressure could drop by 8 to 14 points, which can make a significant difference in your health risks."

— *The Mayo Clinic*

If you're at a high risk of developing high blood pressure due to your ethnicity (African-Americans are in this high-risk group), lifestyle choices (such as smoking and high sodium intake) or weight (obesity is a leading indicator of hypertension risk), the DASH diet is the recommended diet for reducing your risk.

The DASH Diet and Type 2 Diabetes

The DASH diet was rated by *US News & World Report* as the best diet for combating type 2 diabetes, or for people at high risk of developing the disease. It has been shown that the symptoms and severity of type 2 diabetes can be greatly lessened with a DASH-style diet, and that the condition can sometimes even be reversed with these dietary changes.

All of the foods included in the DASH diet are recommended to help improve the health of those with type 2 diabetes, but some are particularly effective. Nuts can improve glucose control in diabetics. Similarly, the high fiber content of the diet works to slow the absorption of sugar, which helps to prevent serious swings in blood sugar levels. The high level of antioxidants in all the DASH-recommended fresh fruits and vegetables can also help to prevent or reduce type 2 diabetes complications.

One of the most important ways that the DASH diet can help those with or at risk for type 2 diabetes is in weight loss. Excess body fat—particularly abdominal fat—is one of the biggest contributors to insulin insensitivity. It also further increases the risk of heart disease for diabetics.

The DASH Diet and Metabolic Syndrome

Metabolic syndrome serves as an umbrella term for a group of obesity- and insulin-related symptoms. The syndrome is commonly referred to as "pre-diabetes" because it often leads to type 2 diabetes if it isn't corrected.

The typical diagnostic markers of metabolic syndrome include a large waist size, high fasting glucose (blood sugar) levels, high triglycerides and elevated HDL cholesterol. All of these negative symptoms can be improved by following the DASH diet. DASH's lowered intake of bad fats and increased intake of good fats and fiber helps to lower HDL cholesterol and triglyceride levels. The nutrients you'll consume on the DASH diet, coupled with significant fat loss around the abdomen, can reverse, prevent or significantly reduce metabolic syndrome.

The DASH Diet and Heart Disease

People with high blood pressure, type 2 diabetes and metabolic syndrome have a high risk of developing heart disease. Since the DASH diet addresses these conditions, it in turn addresses your risk for heart disease.

Even if you are not confronting or have a high risk of developing these conditions, the DASH diet is still an excellent choice. Heart disease is the leading cause of death in America, and health professionals have long known that a diet low in unhealthy fats and high in healthy fats and fiber will positively impact heart health. As a result, the DASH diet has gained the support of the American Heart Association because of its heart-healthy diet.[4]

In addition to the benefits for your heart, the DASH diet has also been credited with lowering the risk of kidney stones and improving digestive and colon health; your heart won't be the only beneficiary of a DASH eating plan!

Fat Intake and Weight Loss

In regard to fat intake and weight loss, the DASH diet:

- **Is far lower in fat than the typical American diet.** Since it is lower in fat, it is also lower in overall calories.
- **Reduces or eliminates unhealthy fats.** Fried foods, fast food, and highly processed foods are excluded or limited.
- **Includes plenty of healthy fats such as unsaturated fats and healthy saturated fats such as Omega-3 fats.** These healthy fats are not only good for your body, but also helpful if you want to lose weight. They're typically found in foods that are lower in calories. Plus, they can help your body rid itself of excess unhealthy body fats.

Fiber Intake and Weight Loss

A diet high in fiber is great for your health and essential to weight loss. The DASH diet is rich in two types of fibers: soluble and insoluble. These fibers help you to feel full, aid in efficient digestion (helping you rid your body of wastes, toxins and fat) and slow the absorption of fat and sugar into your bloodstream. This slowed absorption rate aids in weight loss by:

- Helping your body to regulate and respond to insulin more efficiently, which reduces the risk or symptoms of metabolic syndrome.
- Reducing the amount of excess fat that is stored in the body.

Vitamin C and Weight Loss

Because the DASH diet is so high in fresh fruits and vegetables, you will consume a wide range of essential vitamins, minerals and antioxidants. One of the most important of these nutrients is vitamin C.

In recent years, a great deal of research has come out about the value of vitamin C in weight loss—particularly fat loss. Vitamin C has a two-pronged role in the process of losing excess fat:

- **Vitamin C reduces the effects of stress on the body, which in turn reduces the amount of cortisol (the stress hormone) that is released into the bloodstream.** Cortisol's main function is to aid in the storage of fat around the abdomen as a biological insurance policy against famine. When you reduce the amount of stress in your life, you reduce the amount of cortisol that is released into your system. This means that less of what you eat will end up stored in your abdomen. It also means that your body may start ridding itself of the abdominal fat you already have.

- **Vitamin C is the building block for a compound called L-carnitine.** You can think of L-carnitine as a transporter of stored fat. Once the signal has been sent that you no longer need this fat, it will be turned back into glucose and used as energy. That's where L-carnitine comes in. Our bodies make L-carnitine naturally, but they require a good deal of vitamin C to do so. Vitamin C is a water-soluble vitamin, which means that we don't store much of it at a time and must consume it regularly. Vitamin C is primarily used to fight infection and rebuild cells; any vitamin C that remains after accomplishing these tasks is then allocated toward tasks such as generating L-carnitine. As a result, you need to get plenty of vitamin C on a daily basis if you want it to contribute to weight loss. The foods of the DASH diet deliver this necessary dosage.

Calorie Intake and Weight Loss

For years, the mainstream approach to weight loss was based on a "calories in/calories out" formula: If you take in fewer calories than you burn, you'll lose weight. We now know this is only partially correct. Current research shows that reducing calories *can* result in weight loss, but that the reduction of calories alone will not necessarily result in fat loss.

It is common for people who have lost weight to still appear flabby and out of shape. This is because a diet plan that only involves the reduction of calories can result in the loss of lean muscle tissue and water instead of stored fat; this is particularly the case when calories have been dramatically reduced.

The average American takes in roughly 3000 calories per day, which is more than most people need. Instead of simply advocating a reduction of this amount, however, the DASH diet prescribes a caloric intake that varies from participant to participant. This prescribed intake takes your current weight, weight loss goals, activity level and body type into consideration—a process that is covered in the next section. With this personalized method of setting calorie intakes, the DASH diet not only avoids having so few calories that you risk losing lean muscle tissue instead of fat, but also ensures that you have enough nutrients to support your activity level and speed fat loss.

An All-Around Healthy Plan for Weight Loss Success

The DASH diet incorporates multiple healthy eating strategies, providing a nutritionally sound method of weight loss. With this realistic and delicious healthy eating plan, DASH participants have found that they are more likely to reach their weight loss goals and make a permanent lifestyle change for the better.

IS THE DASH DIET RIGHT FOR YOU?

I f you suffer from high blood pressure or have a high risk of developing blood pressure problems, the DASH diet is an ideal health plan for you. In fact, with its healthy eating methods, the DASH diet is an excellent plan for everyone.

Due to the increasing problem of obesity in the US and elsewhere, metabolic syndrome is also on the rise. If you are significantly overweight and/or have a large waistline and excess abdominal fat, you may have metabolic syndrome or are in danger of developing it.

The good news is that metabolic syndrome can be partially or fully reversed with a combination of exercise and a DASH-style diet. Experts have found that similar results can be achieved for those with type 2 diabetes.

But what if you are not affected by these illnesses? What if you are just looking for a healthy way to lose weight and potentially prevent these conditions later in life?

If you are considering the DASH diet for weight loss and preventative reasons, then you are likely to find it to be an attractive candidate for long-term health. The DASH diet recommends that you eat a wide variety of foods from all of the food groups, guides you through the process of identifying your ideal calorie intake, and often boosts participants' metabolism and energy levels. While many other diets propose unhealthy eating patterns and starvation, DASH's healthy food-centric plan is an excellent and realistic choice for many.

Additional benefits of the DASH diet:

- You are likely to find DASH-friendly food options when eating at restaurants or a friend's house.
- The realistic methods of DASH make it easier to maintain your weight once you've reached your ideal weight.
- You have the option to choose a sodium level that is appropriate for you.
- The DASH diet outlines how you can increase or decrease your caloric intake as your activity level and body mass change.
- It is simple to adapt popular recipes to fit the DASH diet.

It's easy to see why millions of people have considered choosing the DASH diet to improve their health and lose excess weight and fat. With this guide, you'll have everything you need to succeed on the diet.

DASH to a Better Lifestyle

- **Chapter 5:** Planning Your DASH Diet

- **Chapter 6:** Transitioning to the DASH Diet

PLANNING YOUR DASH DIET

G ood preparation is essential to making any new endeavor successful. You need to know that you have the right tools and supplies—and that your goals are realistic—before you get started.

The DASH diet isn't difficult or complicated, but it will likely cause a significant change to your lifestyle. Being successful on the DASH diet requires commitment, determination, and a bit of planning to avoid the pitfalls that might cause discouragement or frustration.

What is Your Body Mass Index?

The first thing that you need to do is establish your health and fitness goals. Most people rely on the bathroom scale to tell them how much weight they need to lose, but that's really not the most accurate measurement.

Start by determining your *body mass index* (BMI). This index approximates the percentage of your body weight that is fat. You can get your body fat calculated by professionals or purchase a body fat measurement kit; alternately, you can get a fairly accurate measurement of your BMI with a measuring tape and an online calculator.

Next, measure your weight. To do this, you'll need to weigh yourself first thing in the morning, after urinating and before eating or drinking. Wear only your underwear or nothing at all. Record your weight in the appropriate blank on the *BMI Assessment Form* at the end of this chapter.

Next, you'll need to gather some measurements to use in calculating your BMI.

For men, you'll measure your neck and abdomen circumference. Be sure the measuring tape keeps in contact with your skin without pulling it too tightly. To measure your abdomen, wrap the measuring tape around your body at a point just below your belly button.

For women, you'll measure the circumference of your neck, waist and hips. Measure your waist at the slimmest point of your torso and measure your hips just below the hip bones; the measuring tape should cross the top portion of your buttocks. As you take these measurements, you can write them down on the *BMI Assessment Form* that is at the end of this chapter.

Once you have your measurements, you can calculate your BMI using one of the many free calculators that are available online. One calculator that you can use is: http://www.linear-software.com/online.html.

If you are using the calculator in the link, the steps to calculate your BMI are:

- Find the section that pertains to your gender (either "Male" or "Female").
- Enter your age and weight.
- Enter your measurements in the "Tape Measurement Method" column.
- Click the "Calculate" button.
- Scroll down to see your results below. Enter the value for your "Body Fat %" on the "Body Fat %" line of the *BMI Assessment Form* that appears at the end of this chapter.

If you use a different calculator, follow the steps necessary to calculate your body fat percentage and enter the value on the "Body Fat %" line of the *BMI Assessment Form* that appears at the end of this chapter.

With an understanding of your body fat percentage, you can begin understanding your current state of health and have a point of comparison after you have started following the DASH diet. While you can weigh yourself along the way and celebrate pounds lost, recalculating your BMI is often a more efficient way to track your progress.

If you follow both the DASH diet and the DASH to Fitness workout plan, you'll likely be gaining lean muscle mass as you lose fat. In this situation, a scale can't tell the difference between muscle weight and fat weight; lean muscle weighs more than fat, but is more compact than fat tissue. As a result, the scale may say you've gained weight, but you are likely to see an improvement in your BMI. To see an example of this improvement in action, you can return to the BMI calculator you used for your initial calculation and reduce your measurements by several inches (just one or two inches at the neck, and a few to several inches at the waist, abdomen or hips). This will show what your BMI would be given those hypothetical measurements.

What is Your Basal Metabolic Rate?

Once you have an understanding of your BMI, it is important to calculate the number of calories that your body requires to maintain your current weight. This calculation will help you understand the number of calories you should consume in order to lose weight at a safe and comfortable pace.

To perform this calculation, you will first calculate your *basal metabolic rate* or BMR. The BMR formula takes your height, weight, age and gender into account in its calculation. This method is likely to be more accurate than calculating your calorie needs based solely on body weight. Since leaner bodies burn more calories than less leaner ones, this method will be accurate unless if you are very muscular or very obese. If you're very fit and muscular, you may need to add more calories, and if you're very overweight you may need to deduct them. Trial and error will help you make these types of adjustments as you progress in your diet.

The following formula will calculate your BMR:

- **For Women**: BMR = 655 + (4.35 x weight in pounds) + (4.7 x height in inches) – (4.7 x age in years)
- **For Men**: BMR = 66 + (6.23 x weight in pounds) + (12.7 x height in inches) – (6.8 x age in year)

Calculate your BMR and record it in on the *BMI Assessment Form* at the end of this chapter.

What Are Your Daily Calorie Requirements?

In order to determine your daily calorie requirements (DCR) you'll need to factor in your activity level. To do this, we use what is known as the *Harris Benedict Equation.*

To determine your total daily calorie needs, multiply your BMR by the appropriate activity factor, as follows:

If you are sedentary (little or no exercise):
Calorie-Calculation = BMR x 1.2

If you are lightly active (sports 1–3 days/week):
Calorie-Calculation = BMR x 1.375

If you are moderately active (sports 3–5 days/week):
Calorie-Calculation = BMR x 1.55

If you are very active (sports 6–7 days a week):
Calorie-Calculation = BMR x 1.725

If you are extra active (sports & physical job or 2x training):
Calorie-Calculation = BMR x 1.9

Calculate your BMR and record it on the *BMI Assessment Form* at the end of this chapter.

Once you know the number of calories needed to maintain your weight, you can easily calculate the number of calories you need to eat in order to gain or lose weight:

One pound equals 3500 calories, so to lose one pound a week you would deduct 500 calories from your total daily caloric requirements (not your BMR). To lose two pounds a week, you would need to deduct 1000 calories per day.

For people whose daily caloric requirement is low, trying to lose weight solely by cutting calories may be impractical and unsustainable. It's healthy to combine increased activity and decreased calorie intake, but this is especially true for those who already have a low calorie requirement.

You can start out using the caloric requirements for your present activity level, minus 500–1000 calories per day. In two weeks, if you're staying on schedule with your DASH to Fitness plan, recalculate your daily calorie needs using the appropriate new activity level. This will ensure that you're getting enough nutrition yet still staying on track for your weight loss.

The **DASH Diet Health Plan** *does not recommend cutting calories below 1500 per day for women and 1800 per day for men.*

BMI Assessment Form

Date _____

Weight _____

Neck _____

Waist _____ *(Women)*

Hips _____ *(Women)*

Abdomen _____ *(Men)*

Body Fat % _____

BMR: _____ calories

DCR: _____

Note: You might want to copy several blank assessment forms to help track your progress until you reach your goals.

6

TRANSITIONING TO THE DASH DIET

The decision to take on a new diet plan is difficult, one that will require discipline and hard work. Once you commit to incorporating the DASH diet into your lifestyle, it is essential to properly prepare for your journey towards health.

Here are some steps and tips that you should integrate into your lifestyle at least one week before you officially start the DASH diet.

Clean House

Changing your eating habits is a challenging task, so it's best to eliminate temptations that might jeopardize your health. One of the best things you can do to achieve success is to eliminate all of the off-limits foods from the house.

Get rid of processed foods (prepared snack foods, chips, fried foods, etc.), as well as high-sodium and high-fat condiments such as salad dressings, soy sauces, etc. You know your own weaknesses better than anyone, so even if something is allowed on the DASH diet food list, get rid of it if you know it is an item you will have a hard time consuming in moderation.

Plan Your Menu Ahead of Time

The key to achieving success with the DASH diet is to plan your meals in advance. Whether you use the menu plans provided in the book or create your own, it helps to know ahead of time what you'll be eating the first couple of weeks. Preparation of meal plans helps with shopping, prepares you for a new way of eating, and eliminates unhealthy snacking once you begin the diet.

Prepare Your Taste Buds

The week before you start your diet, start to cut back on portion sizes, take the saltshaker off the table, opt for fruit when it comes to dessert, and skip the junk food. Focus on these initial steps, without having to worry about calories or any of the other aspects of the DASH diet. By the time you start your diet, your body will already be in the process of adjusting to the new way of eating (and intense cravings will have diminished).

Start Your Exercise Plan a Week Early or a Week Late

Starting a new diet and a new workout program at the same time can be overwhelming. If you thrive on that kind of radical change, then go ahead and do it. If not, start your exercise plan the week before or the week after you start the DASH diet. Preparing for the DASH diet is not about results; the point is to make the transition as easy as possible. One week won't make a significant difference in your health plan, but it can be the difference between motivation and frustration.

The Top 10 Tips to Prepare for Success

1. Trade your saltshaker for salt substitute

Plan ahead and eliminate salt whenever you can, so that you can enjoy it in other foods where it cannot be eliminated. This is especially important if you have high blood pressure and need to follow the lowest sodium version of the diet. When possible, use salt substitutes or another herb blend in place of salt.

2. Make the right choices the easiest ones

Make sure that fresh fruits and other healthy snacks are more visible than tempting treats such as dark chocolate and sorbet. To ward off temptation, keep healthy snacks and a water bottle accessible, and avoid the fast-food lunch trap by bringing your own meals to work.

3. Exercise first thing in the morning

Something always gets in the way of exercise, especially when a new workout routine is being initiated. Until you're hooked on fitness, and not inclined to use any excuse that comes your way, it is best to work out as soon as you wake up. It is always possible to change your workout schedule, but wait until working out has become a habit. (Usually, this takes about thirty days.)

4. Drink a ton of water

Most experts recommend drinking at least sixty four ounces of water per day. If you're not already doing this, you need to start. Your new diet is full of foods that aid digestion, but you need a lot of water to get things moving. Adequate water will also help you to lose excess stored water, feel fuller longer and have more energy.

5. Skip the restaurants for the first two weeks

While you shouldn't deprive yourself of things you enjoy, like going out to eat, it's better to wait until you're used to making healthier choices, and seeing results that motivate you to stick with the diet. If you go out to eat before your healthy choices become second nature, you may accidentally sabotage yourself. One breadbasket won't set you back physically, but it may do damage to your resolve. Most dieters are familiar with the anger and frustration that follows a binge or even a misstep. You need to feel good about yourself and your progress, so limit opportunities that put you off course.

6. Buddy-up, or get your friends to support you

If possible, enlist a family member or friend to go on the diet with you. Getting someone to join you for workouts can also be a big help. Accountability and mutual motivation is an important factor in sticking with your plan. If you don't have anyone who wants to diet or work out with you, at least let your friends and family know how important your goals are to you, and don't be afraid to ask them to help remove temptation and keep you on course.

7. Enjoy eating

The menu plans and recipes in this book are tools to guide you and help you follow the DASH diet. They are not, however, set in stone. Feel free to create your own menu plans using the foods list, your daily servings guide, and any of the thousands of DASH-friendly recipes available. If you're not enjoying your food, you won't be on the diet for very long.

8. Keep a journal

Keep a small notebook handy and jot down your progress. Write down what you eat and how you feel after: eating a healthy meal, a good work-out, or winning a battle against temptation. These notes can really help keep you motivated, especially when you hit a rough patch.

9. Avoid or plan for food triggers

Most people have certain triggers that result in overeating or making poor food choices. Identify your triggers and figure out ways to avoid them altogether, or at least to outwit them. If watching TV isn't the same without snacks, then have plenty of healthy ones on hand, or eliminate TV for the first couple of weeks. Bad habits are easier to avoid once the habit-inducing trigger is recognized.

10. Circumvent stress eating

Stress-induced eating is a common problem. It's easy to justify eating during stressful moments, which is why it is important to develop an emergency plan of action before you face the situation. Identify stress-alleviating alternatives in advance, such as going on a short walk or calling a good friend, and follow through with the plan when you rec-ognize your stress levels rise.

Laughter and exercise both release endorphins, which soothe and alleviate feelings of stress. It takes only about ten to fifteen minutes for you to start feeling the effects, and both activities will also burn a few extra calories for you. It's a win-win.

Your DASH Diet Eating Plan

- **Chapter 7**: Calorie Requirements & Food Guide

- **Chapter 8**: The DASH Diet Foods & Shopping Guide

- **Chapter 9**: The DASH Diet Menu Plans

CALORIE REQUIREMENTS & FOOD GUIDE

Calorie Requirements

The menu plans included in this book are based on a 2000-calorie diet. If you require more or less calories, we'll show you how to make adjustments while ensuring that you get all the nutrients you need.

The foods chosen for the diet and for the menu plans were selected for their nutrient content, not just their calories. Keep in mind that you need plenty of potassium, magnesium and calcium—be sure to choose foods rich in these micronutrients. Don't forget: the menu plans are a guideline. Choose a plan that is sustainable, and works best for you.

Food Group	Servings Per Day			Serving Size
	1,600 Calories	2,000 Calories	2,600 Calories	
Grains & grain products*	6	6–8	10–11	1 slice bread 1 ounce dry cereal** ½ cup cooked rice, pasta or cereal
Vegetables	3–4	4–5	5–6	1 cup raw leafy vegetable ½ cup cut-up raw or cooked vegetable ½ cup vegetable juice
Fruits	4	4–5	5–6	½ cup fruit juice 1 medium fruit ¼ cup dried fruit ½ cup fresh, frozen or canned fruit
Fat free or low-fat milk and milk products	2–3	2–3	3	1 cup milk or yogurt 1 ½ ounces cheese
Lean meats, poultry, and fish	3–4 or less	6 or less	6 or less	1 ounce cooked meats, poultry or fish 1 egg***
Nuts, seeds, and dry beans	3–4 per week	4–5 per week	1	⅓ cup or 1 ½ ounce nuts 2 tablespoons peanut butter 2 tablespoon or ½ ounce seeds ½ cup cooked legumes
Fats & oils****	2	2–3	3	1 teaspoon soft margarine 1 teaspoon vegetable oil 1 tablespoon mayonnaise 2 tablespoons salad dressing
Sweets and added sugars	3 or less per week	5 or less per week	≤2	1 tablespoon sugar 1 tablespoon jelly or jam ½ cup sorbet, gelatin 1 cup lemonade

Fig. 7.1. Use the chart to plan your menus or help guide you through the aisles when you go grocery shopping.

(Table courtesy of the National Heart, Lung and Blood Institute.)

* Whole grains are recommended as a good source of fiber and nutrients.

** Serving sizes vary between ½ cup–1¼ cups. Check the product's Nutrition Facts label.

*** Since eggs are high in cholesterol, limit egg yolk intake to no more than four per week; two eggs have the same protein content as 1 ounce of meat.

**** Fat content changes serving counts for fats and oils: As an example, 1 tablespoon of regular salad dressing equals 1 serving; 1 tablespoon of a low-fat dressing equals ½ serving; 1 tablespoon of a fat-free dressing equals 0 servings.

THE DASH DIET FOODS & SHOPPING GUIDE

The DASH Diet Foods

Meats and Seafood

Allowed:

- All fish, especially salmon, haddock, mackerel, sardines and other oily fish
- All shellfish
- Beef: lean steaks and roasts, leanest possible ground meat
- Chicken, skinless
- Eggs
- Game birds
- Game meats
- Ground turkey breast
- Lamb: lean stew meat, steaks and roasts
- Pork: lean steaks and roasts
- Turkey, skinless
- Venison

Not Allowed:

- Bacon, except for low-salt turkey bacon

- Jerky
- Packaged cold cuts and deli meats
- Sausage

Dairy

Allowed:
- Almond milk
- Blue cheese
- Cheddar cheese (reduced fat)
- Cow's milk (one percent or nonfat)
- Cream cheese (reduced fat)
- Feta cheese
- Greek yogurt
- Low-fat cottage cheese (or nonfat)
- Margarine or butter substitute
- Mozzarella cheese
- Parmesan cheese (high sodium, so limit quantities)
- Provolone cheese (reduced fat)
- Regular yogurt (low or nonfat)
- Ricotta cheese (reduced fat)
- Sour cream (reduced or nonfat)
- Soy milk
- Swiss cheese

Not Allowed:
- Any full-fat dairy products
- Butter
- Cream

Low-Glycemic Vegetables

Allowed:

- Artichoke
- Arugula
- Asparagus
- Avocado
- Bell peppers
- Broccoli
- Brussels sprouts
- Cabbage
- Cauliflower
- Celery
- Collard greens
- Cucumbers
- Eggplant
- Green beans
- Kale
- Lettuce, preferably Romaine or dark leafy varieties
- Mushrooms
- Mustard greens
- Onions
- Radishes
- Spinach
- Sprouts
- Swiss chard
- Snow peas
- Summer squash
- Turnip greens
- Zucchini

High-Glycemic Vegetables

Allowed:
- Acorn squash
- Butternut squash
- Carrots
- Chickpeas
- English peas
- Spaghetti squash
- Sweet potatoes
- Tomatoes

Very Limited Quantities *(One serving per week)*
- Corn
- White potatoes

Low-Glycemic Fruits

Allowed:
- Apples
- Blackberries
- Blueberries
- Cantaloupe
- Casaba melon
- Cranberries
- Guava
- Honeydew melon
- Lemons
- Limes
- Nectarines
- Papaya
- Peaches

- Raspberries
- Rhubarb
- Strawberries
- Watermelon

High-Glycemic Fruits

Allowed:

- Cherries
- Figs
- Grapefruit
- Kiwi
- Mango
- Oranges
- Pears
- Plums
- Tangerines
- Watermelon

Fats

Allowed:

- Almonds
- Black walnuts
- Brazil nuts
- Canola oil
- Flax seed oil
- Margarine or butter substitute
- Mayonnaise (low fat)
- Olive oil

- Olives (low sodium)
- Sesame seeds
- Sunflower seeds

Not Allowed:
- All other vegetable oils
- Peanut oil
- Sesame oil

Grains

Allowed:
- Almond flour
- Coconut flour
- Wheat germ
- Whole grain, low carb cold cereal
- Whole grain, mixed grain hot cereal
- Whole grain, steel cut oats
- Whole grain bread, preferably very dense
- Whole grain pita
- Whole grain thin style bagels
- Whole grain thin style English muffins
- Whole grain tortillas
- Whole wheat flour

Not Allowed:
- Corn meal
- Corn muffins or cornbread
- Instant or flavored oatmeal
- Sweetened cold cereals

Condiments, Seasonings, and Miscellaneous

Allowed:

- Almond butter
- Caesar dressing
- Coffee
- Dressings (low sodium or no sodium)
- Flax seed or flax seed oil
- Herbs and spices
- Hot sauce
- Iced tea
- Mustard (except honey mustard)
- Peanut butter (in limited quantities)
- Preserves and jellies (no or low sugar)
- Psyllium husk
- Salsa
- Sesame butter (tahini)
- Sour or dill pickles
- Soy sauce (low sodium)
- Tea
- Teriyaki sauce (low sodium)
- Tomato or spaghetti sauce (no sugar added)
- Vegetable, chicken or beef broth (no or low sodium)
- Vinaigrette
- Whey or soy protein powder (no sugar added)

Not Allowed:

- Mayonnaise (full fat)
- Prepared Alfredo or cheese sauce
- Prepared gravy
- Regular commercial salad dressings
- Regular sodium steak, barbecue and other sauces

Sweets

Allowed:
- 1-ounce dark chocolate
- Dried fruits (preferably no sugar added)
- Fudge pops (fat free)
- Frozen fruit bar (no sugar added)
- Gelatin
- Ice cream (low fat)
- Popsicles
- Pudding or pudding cups (fat free)
- Sorbet or sherbet

The DASH Diet Shopping Guide

When you are on a diet, grocery shopping can be a challenging task. Here are a few tips to help make your grocery shopping easier and more nutritious.

Shop Around the Edges of the Store

Buy the majority of your foods from the fresh food sections, which are normally located around the edges of the store. This includes fresh fruits and vegetables, fresh meats, seafood, poultry and fresh dairy products.

Skip the Danger Zones

Stay out of the aisles where processed snacks, such as chips and cookies, are located. Out of sight, out of mind.

Read Your Labels

Don't assume that something is low in sodium just because it isn't salty. Read the labels on everything. It's always best to make your food from scratch so that you can control the sodium content, but that isn't possible for everyone. When you need to buy prepared foods, buy those that are lowest in sodium, sugar and saturated fat. Make note of the best brands so you can eventually shop without having to do any heavy reading.

Buy the Rainbow

To ensure a high intake of antioxidants and micronutrients, choose different kinds of produce every time you shop. Don't just buy green peppers—buy red or orange peppers. Choose lots of dark, leafy greens. Buy fruits that are rich in color, such as watermelon, mango and dark berries. Consuming a diverse variety of produce will help increase each bite's nutritional value.

Choose Your Meat and Seafood Wisely

Whenever possible, buy organic, grass-fed or pasture-raised meats and wild seafood; they have more Omega-3 fats and are more likely to be free of hormones and preservatives. Always choose the leanest cuts of whatever you're buying, and trim visible fat after cooking.

Choose Low-Fat Dairy

Low-fat dairy products should be chosen whenever possible. Cheeses should be nonfat or partially nonfat. Milk should be nonfat or one percent fat. Yogurt should be nonfat and low in sugar or sugar-free.

THE DASH DIET MENU PLANS

This chapter includes a 14-day menu planner to help you get started. Following the menu plans will help you get accustomed to proper portion sizes, new flavors and combinations of healthy foods.

Feel free to substitute the menu plans for your own recipes. Just be mindful of the calories, fat and sodium in the recipes you use, so that you can adjust other meals if needed.

The following menu plans are for a 2000-calorie diet allowing 1500 mg of sodium daily. The actual menus run between 1700–1800 calories to allow for extra snacks of fruit, extra helpings of veggies or an extra beverage of milk or juice.

If you need to adjust your calories up or down, follow the tips provided earlier. For instance, to adjust from a 2000-calorie plan to a 1600-calorie plan then decrease your servings of grains and fruits by one or two each. If you need to increase your calories, increase your fruits and vegetables first, then grains.

If you don't need to keep the sodium intake to a lower level, you can be more liberal with table salt and use more condiments, such as teriyaki sauce or prepared salad dressings.

The only beverages specified on the menu plans are milk and juice. You're free to have water and sweetened or unsweetened hot tea and coffee at every meal. If you have more leeway in your calories, feel free to add fruit juice or milk to a meal.

NOTE: Dishes marked with [*] are recipes provided in your DASH Diet Cookbook.

Menu Plans for Days 1–14

Day 1:

Breakfast:

- 2 scrambled eggs
- ½ cup cantaloupe
- 1 slice whole wheat toast with jam
- 8 ounces nonfat or one percent milk

Snack:

- ¼ cup raw almonds or walnuts
- 1 (6-ounce) vanilla yogurt
- ½ cup blueberries

Lunch:

- Spinach salad with mushrooms and tomatoes
- 1 tablespoon low-fat salad dressing
- 1 sliced chicken breast
- 1 medium orange

Dinner:

- Southwestern Stuffed Peppers [*]
- 1 cup oven-roasted carrots
- 1 whole wheat roll

Dessert:

- 1 cup watermelon

Day 2:

Breakfast:
- Pineapple Banana Breakfast Bowl [*]
- ½ cup cottage cheese

Snack:
- 10 low-sodium crackers
- 4 ounces nonfat cheese
- 1 medium apple

Lunch:
- Whole wheat wrap with 2 slices turkey breast, 1 slice Swiss cheese, ½ cup romaine lettuce, and mustard
- 1 cup low-sodium chicken broth
- ½ cup sliced strawberries

Dinner:
- 1 fillet broiled cod or other fish
- 1 cup steamed spinach
- ½ baked sweet potato with margarine or salt substitute
- 1 cup brown rice

Dessert:
- 1 unsweetened frozen fruit bar

Day 3:

Breakfast:
- ½ cup whole grain cereal
- ¼ cup nonfat or one percent milk
- ½ cup strawberries
- 1 medium banana

Snack:
- 1 sliced tomato with low-sodium salad dressing
- 1 stick string cheese

Lunch:
- New York Turkey Melt [*]
- Salad with spring greens, red onion, and 1 tablespoon low-sodium dressing

Dinner:
- 1 broiled chicken breast with herbs
- 1 cup green beans with 1 teaspoon margarine or olive oil
- 1 cup steamed quinoa with olive oil and pepper

Dessert:
- 1 medium pear

Day 4:

Breakfast:
- 2 egg omelet with ½ cup spinach and ¼ cup sliced mushrooms
- 1 slice whole wheat toast with 1 tablespoon jam
- 6-ounce glass orange juice

Snack:
- ½ cup cottage cheese with ½ cup peaches

Lunch:
- Grilled chicken salad with 1 chicken breast, sliced, and ½ cup each of spinach, tomatoes, and onions
- 1 tablespoon vinaigrette
- 1 medium apple

Dinner:
- Hawaiian Chicken [*]
- 1 cup brown rice
- 1 sliced tomato

Dessert:
- 1 nonfat pudding cup

Day 5:

Breakfast:
- Italian Toast Plate [*]
- 6-ounce glass grapefruit juice

Snack:
- Fruit salad with ½ cup cantaloupe and ½ cup pineapple
- ¼ cup sunflower seeds (unsalted)

Lunch:
- 1 cup low-sodium tomato soup (made with nonfat milk)
- 10 low-sodium crackers
- 1 medium banana

Dinner:
- ½ pound boiled or steamed shrimp with cocktail sauce
- 1 cup sautéed kale with olive oil and salt substitute
- 1 cup roasted carrots with olive oil and salt substitute
- ½ cup brown rice

Dessert:
- 1 large slice honeydew melon

Day 6:

Breakfast:
- Tomato Cheddar Omelet [*]
- ½ whole wheat bagel with 1 tablespoon jam
- ½ cup sliced pears

Snack:
- 1 (6-ounce) cup yogurt
- 1 medium orange

Lunch:
- Chicken breast sandwich on whole wheat pita with 2 slices tomato, sliced onion and ½ cup lettuce
- 1 tablespoon low-fat mayo
- 1 medium banana

Dinner:
- 1 fillet baked or broiled salmon
- 1 cup steamed cauliflower with 1 tablespoon margarine or olive oil
- ½ cup sautéed mushrooms and onions
- 6 spears roasted asparagus with olive oil and pepper

Dessert:
- 1 low-fat fudge popsicle

Day 7:

Breakfast:
- Smoothie with 6-ounce vanilla yogurt, 1 banana and 1 tablespoon cocoa powder
- ½ red grapefruit
- ¼ cup almonds

Snack:
- 1 stick low-fat or nonfat string cheese
- 1 cup honeydew melon

Lunch:
- Salad with 6 shrimp, 1 cup romaine lettuce, ½ cup tomato, and ½ cup red pepper
- 1 tablespoon balsamic vinaigrette
- 1 slice whole wheat toast with margarine

Dinner:
- Artichoke, Shrimp & Scallops [*]
- 1 cup sautéed Swiss chard

Dessert:
- 1-ounce square dark chocolate

Day 8:

Breakfast:
- Cherry French Toast [*]
- 6-ounce glass milk

Snack:
- ½ cup cottage cheese
- ½ cup pineapple
- ¼ cup blueberries

Lunch:
- 1 cup low-sodium vegetable soup
- ½ whole wheat bagel
- 1 tablespoon nonfat cream cheese
- 1 medium apple

Dinner:
- 1 cup whole wheat angel hair pasta
- ½ cup spaghetti sauce
- 1 tablespoon Parmesan cheese
- Spinach salad with onions, mushrooms, and red peppers
- 1 tablespoon low-fat Italian dressing

Dessert:
- ½ cup low-fat ice cream

Day 9:

Breakfast:
- 2 scrambled eggs
- 2 slices low-salt turkey bacon
- 1 cup grapes
- 1 slice whole wheat toast with 1 tablespoon margarine

Snack:
- ½ cup dried apricots
- ¼ cup pumpkin seeds

Lunch:
- Loaded Turkey Sandwich [*]
- 1 cup mixed fresh berries

Dinner:
- 6-ounce lean pork tenderloin
- 1 cup steamed broccoli with 1 tablespoon olive oil and pepper
- ½ baked acorn squash with 1 tablespoon olive oil or margarine
- ½ cup applesauce

Dessert:
- 1 cup roasted fresh pineapple

Day 10:

Breakfast:
- Bacon-Avocado Egg Dish [*]
- ½ red grapefruit
- 6-ounce glass milk

Snack:
- 1 medium banana spread with 1 tablespoon low-salt peanut butter

Lunch:
- 6-ounce hamburger patty
- ½ cup sautéed mushrooms and onions
- 1 whole wheat bun
- 1 cup steamed green beans

Dinner:
- 6-ounce broiled chicken breast
- 1 cup roasted zucchini and peppers with 1 tablespoon olive oil and herbs
- 1 cup steamed carrots with 1 tablespoon olive oil and salt substitute

Dessert:
- 1 nonfat pudding cup

Day 11:

Breakfast:
- 1 cup steel-cut oats
- ½ cup one percent milk
- ¼ cup dried cranberries
- 1 tablespoon honey
- 6-ounce glass orange juice

Snack:
- 5 low-sodium crackers
- 1 tablespoon peanut butter
- 1 pear

Lunch:
- 1 cup low-sodium minestrone
- 1 whole wheat pita with 1 slice mozzarella, 1 slice cold roast beef, ½ cup tomato, and 1 tablespoon low-sodium Italian dressing
- 1 medium mango

Dinner:
- Honey Mustard Chicken [*]
- 1 cup baked Hubbard squash with 1 tablespoon olive oil and nutmeg
- 1 cup steamed cauliflower with 1 tablespoon olive oil and pepper

Dessert:
- 1 popsicle

Day 12:

Breakfast:
- Blackberry Quinoa Bowl [*]
- 1 boiled egg

Snack:
- 2 slices roast beef
- 2 slices Swiss cheese
- 6 whole wheat low-sodium crackers

Lunch:
- 1 cup cottage cheese
- ½ cup blueberries
- ½ cup fresh peaches

Dinner:
- 1 cup shrimp stir-fry with 6 shrimp and ¼ cup each of carrots, sprouts, onion and mushrooms (1 tablespoon canola oil and 1 tablespoon low-sodium soy sauce)
- 1 cup brown rice

Dessert:
- ½ cup sorbet

Day 13:

Breakfast:
- ½ cup whole grain cold cereal
- 1 medium sliced banana
- ¼ cup one percent milk
- 6-ounce glass orange juice

Snack:
- 6-ounce cup yogurt
- ¼ cup walnuts

Lunch:
- Shrimp Kebabs [*]
- ½ cup quinoa

Dinner:
- 6 ounce lean broiled steak
- 1 tablespoon steak sauce, low-sodium
- 1 cup roasted Brussels sprouts
- ½ cup steamed summer squash with 1 tablespoon olive oil

Dessert:
- 1 baked apple with 1 teaspoon honey and 1 teaspoon nutmeg

Day 14:

Breakfast:
- ½ cup low-sodium granola
- ¼ cup one percent milk
- ½ cup sliced strawberries

Snack:
- 5 low-sodium crackers
- 2 slices Swiss cheese

Lunch:
- 1 wheat tortilla with 3-ounce sliced steak
- ¼ cup sliced onion
- ¼ cup diced tomato
- 1 tablespoon low-sodium dressing
- 1 cup grapes

Dinner:
- 1 cup frozen cheese ravioli
- ½ cup marinara sauce
- 1 cup steamed broccoli with 1 tablespoon olive oil and salt substitute
- 1 cup roasted butternut squash with nutmeg and 1 tablespoon olive oil

Dessert:
- 1 cup nonfat pudding

A Sample Menu for Busy Workdays

Breakfast

- ½ cup hot granola with ¼ cup one percent milk
- 1 banana

or

- Peach smoothie with 6 ounces peach yogurt, ½ cup blueberries, and ¼ cup nonfat milk

Snack:

- 1 banana
- ¼ cup unsalted almonds

Lunch:

- 1 cup Italian vegetable soup
- 6 whole wheat crackers
- 2 slices provolone cheese

or

- Roast beef sandwich on whole wheat toast with sliced tomato and 1 tablespoon low-sodium dressing

Dinner:

- Snapper fillet broiled with herbs and olive oil
- 1 cup steamed Brussels sprouts with 1 tablespoon olive oil
- 1 cup brown rice with 1 tablespoon margarine

or

- 1 cup penne pasta with ¼ cup pesto sauce
- Spinach salad with mushrooms, onions, and sliced oranges

Dessert:

- ½ cup sorbet

or

- 1-ounce square dark chocolate

A Sample Menu for Weekends

Breakfast:
- 2 scrambled eggs
- 1 slice whole wheat toast with 1 tablespoon jam
- ½ cup cantaloupe

or

- 1 slice French toast with 1 tablespoon margarine and 1 tablespoon pancake syrup
- 2 slices turkey bacon
- 1 medium orange

Snack:
- 1 cup fresh pineapple

or

- 2 stalks celery with 1 tablespoon low-fat cream cheese

Lunch:
- 1 cup low-sodium tomato soup
- 1 slice wheat bread with 1 slice mozzarella, broiled

or

- Chicken breast salad with 1 cup spinach, red peppers, sliced oranges, and onions and 1 tablespoon poppy seed dressing

Dinner:
- 1 cup brown rice with roasted winter squash and mushrooms
- 1 thin broiled pork chop
- 1 cup sautéed kale

or

- 6-ounce lean steak
- 1 cup roasted summer squash with onions
- ½ baked sweet potato with 1 tablespoon margarine

Dessert:

- 1 low-fat pudding cup

or

- 1 cup fresh mango

A Sample Menu for Entertaining

Breakfast:
- Huevos Rancheros [*]
- Baked apple
- 6-ounce glass orange juice

or

- Spinach omelet with low-fat ricotta cheese, spinach, onion, and red pepper
- 1 slice whole wheat toast with 1 tablespoon honey

Snack:
- Low-salt popcorn with olive oil and garlic powder

or

- Cucumber spears with smoked salmon and cream cheese

Lunch:
- Raspberry Spinach Salad [*]
- Whole wheat roll

or

- Grilled Chicken and Fruit Plate [*]

Dinner:
- Peel and eat shrimp (⅓ pound per serving)
- Grilled zucchini wedges
- Roasted carrots
- Artichokes with 1 tablespoon white wine vinaigrette

or

- Baked salmon with rosemary
- Mashed cauliflower with olive oil and pepper
- Maple-glazed baked acorn squash

Dessert:

- Raspberry sorbet

or

- Low-fat chocolate mousse

DASH to Fitness

- **Chapter 10:** Your 28-Day DASH to Fitness Workout Plan

YOUR 28-DAY DASH TO FITNESS WORKOUT PLAN

About the DASH to Fitness Workout Plan

Customize the 28-Day DASH to Fitness Workout Plan based on what is available to you, your likes and dislikes and any injuries or limitations.

The DASH to Fitness Plan includes both cardio and strength training. There are two choices for you when planning your own individual program:

- The Alternating Plan
- The Combo Plan

On the Alternating Plan, there are three days dedicated to cardio, with strength training on the three alternating days. For example, you might do cardio Monday, Wednesday and Friday and strength training Tuesday, Thursday and Saturday. The days you choose are up to you, but they do need to alternate. Each workout takes thirty minutes.

On the Combo Plan, you do strength training and cardio on the same day, six days per week. You'll alternate between lower body strength training and upper body strength training (each three times per week). The Combo Plan is also comprised of thirty-minute workouts and is generally a bit more difficult for beginners, so if you haven't worked out in some time, it might be easier for you to start with the Alternating Plan.

You're more than welcome to change routines after the initial twenty-eight days; in fact, we recommend it. Our bodies become accustomed to workouts after twenty-one to thirty days. By changing the type or intensity of the workout you can keep your metabolism running on high and usually avoid any plateaus.

If you choose swimming for your cardio the first twenty-eight days, you might want to try walking for the next four weeks. If you choose the Alternating Plan for the first twenty-eight days, you may want to do the Combo Plan the next month.

Whichever workout plan you choose, you'll be doing interval training, both for cardio and during strength training. Interval training is simply alternating short segments of harder work in between longer segments of moderate work. Interval training is an effective method of building lean muscle and burning fat. It's great for your cardiovascular system, revs up your metabolism, and gets results fast.

Keep in mind that our bodies respond to the level of work they're used to. If you've been sedentary for some time, your body will respond quickly to fast walking. For someone who has been exercising regularly for some time, they'd have to run or walk on a steep incline to get the same results.

Getting Started with the Workout Plans

These workouts are designed so that anyone can do them, without any equipment other than a good pair of athletic shoes. However, if you are completely new to working out and need instruction for specific stretches and the weight training moves, there are plenty of books, websites, and DVDs that can help.

If you are extremely overweight or out of shape you may want to start out with steady-paced cardio and strength training. Simply do your cardio at a moderate pace for the entire workout and skip the cardio segments in between strength training moves. After a month or two, ask your doctor about incorporating one of the interval training programs.

If you want to increase the intensity of your workouts, there are a few ways to do so:

- For cardio, you can increase the length of your intense segments and decrease the length of your moderate segments.
- You can also increase the incline on your treadmill, choose a steeper path for outdoor walking, choose a more difficult stroke for swimming or carry small weights when you're walking.
- In strength training, lift slowly for increased intensity, or increase the number of reps you do.

The Combo Workout Plans

The Combo Workout Plans incorporate both cardio and strength training into a thirty-minute workout. You'll do the same cardio workout each day, six days a week, choosing from the walking, running, biking or swimming plans.

You'll do the lower body strength training routine and the upper body strength training routine on alternate days. (Both of these include some abdominal exercises, since you can safely and effectively work your abs without a day of rest in between sessions.)

When you're doing the Combo Workout Plans, it's best to start with cardio. The goal of resistance training workout is muscle fatigue. Strength training is what builds lean muscle fast, but it isn't a good idea to exhaust your muscles right before you head out for a run.

If you're doing your cardio outdoors and strength training at home, don't worry about the downtime in between. Contrary to traditional thought, you don't need do thirty minutes of uninterrupted exercise to reap the benefits.

Cardio

Cardio Workout for Walking Outdoors

2 Minutes: Stretch and warm up. Be sure to stretch your neck, shoulders, arms, back and legs.

4 Minutes: Walk at a moderate pace.

2 Minutes: Walk at a fast pace, fast enough to prevent easy conversation.

4 Minutes: Walk at a moderate pace.

2 Minutes: Walk at a fast pace.

4 Minutes: Walk at a moderate pace.

2 Minutes: Cool down by repeating your stretching exercises.

Cardio Workout for Walking or Running on a Treadmill

2 Minutes: Stretch and warm up.

4 Minutes: Walk/run at a moderate pace or on flat terrain.

2 Minutes: Walk/run at a fast pace or on an incline.

4 Minutes: Walk/run at a moderate pace or on flat terrain.

2 Minutes: Walk/run at a fast pace or on an incline.

4 Minutes: Walk/run at a moderate pace or on flat terrain.

2 Minutes: Cool down by repeating your stretching exercises.

Cardio Workout for Running Outdoors (Recommended only for those already accustomed to running regularly)

2 Minutes: Stretch and warm up.

4 Minutes: Run at a moderate pace on flat terrain.

2 Minutes: Run sprints or up and down stairs.

4 Minutes: Run at a moderate pace.

2 Minutes: Run sprints or up and down stairs.

4 Minutes: Run at a moderate pace.

2 Minutes: Cool down by repeating stretching exercises.

Cardio Workout for Cycling (Indoors or Outdoors)

2 Minutes: Stretch and warm up.

4 Minutes: Cycle at a moderate pace or low resistance.

2 Minutes: Cycle at a fast pace or higher resistance.

4 Minutes: Cycle at a moderate pace or low resistance.

2 Minutes: Cycle at a fast pace or higher resistance.

4 Minutes: Cycle at a moderate pace or low resistance.

2 Minutes: Cool down by repeating stretching exercises.

Cardio Workout for Swimming

2 Minutes: Stretch and warm up (in or out of the water).

4 Minutes: Swim at a moderate pace using the crawl stroke.

2 Minutes: Swim at a faster pace or using the butterfly stroke.

4 Minutes: Swim at a moderate pace using the crawl stroke.

2 Minutes: Swim at a faster pace or using the butterfly stroke.

4 Minutes: Swim at a moderate pace using the crawl stroke.

2 Minutes: Cool down by repeating stretching exercises.

Lower Body Strength Training Routine

1 Minute: Warm up by stretching.

Do twenty front lunges, alternating legs five lunges at a time. (In other words, do five lunges with your left leg, then five lunges with your right, until you have completed a total of twenty lunges.)

1 Minute: Run in place, jump rope or do jumping jacks.

Do ten squats.

1 Minute: Run in place, jump rope or do jumping jacks.

Do twenty hamstring lifts.

1 Minute: Run in place, jump rope or do jumping jacks.

Do twenty leg lifts or reverse crunches.

1 Minute: Run in place, jump rope or do jumping jacks.

Do twenty modified crunches (lifting only until your shoulders leave the floor).

1 Minute: Cool down by repeating stretching exercises.

Upper Body Strength Training Routine

1 Minute: Warm up by stretching.

Do twenty push-ups. (If doing full body pushups is too difficult, start on your knees with ankles crossed.)

1 Minute: Run in place, jump rope or do jumping jacks.

Do twenty seated chair dips.

1 Minute: Run in place, jump rope or do jumping jacks.

Do twenty alternating crunches (aka oblique or scissor crunches).

1 Minute: Run in place, jump rope or do jumping jacks.

1 Minute: Cool down by repeating stretching exercises.

The Alternating Workout Plans

The Alternating Workout Plans use the same moves and steps as the Combo Plans—you're simply combining workouts and doing them on alternating days. Three days per week you'll do your cardio workout, the other three days you'll do a combined strength-training workout.

Cardio

To do the thirty-minute cardio workout, simply choose your preferred method of cardio from the Combo Plans and double the number of segments, with the exception of the warm-up and cool down times.

Strength Training Routine

2 Minutes: Warm up by stretching.

Do twenty front lunges, alternating legs five lunges at a time.

1 Minute: Run in place, jump rope or do jumping jacks.

Do ten squats.

1 Minute: Run in place, jump rope or do jumping jacks.

Do twenty hamstring lifts (aka toe raises).

1 Minute: Run in place, jump rope or do jumping jacks.

Do twenty leg lifts or reverse crunches.

1 Minute: Run in place, jump rope or do jumping jacks.

Do twenty modified crunches (lifting only until shoulders leave the floor).

1 Minute: Run in place, jump rope or do jumping jacks.

Do twenty alternating crunches (aka oblique or scissor crunches).

1 Minute: Run in place, jump rope or do jumping jacks.

Do twenty push-ups. (If full body pushups are too difficult, start on your knees with ankles crossed.)

1 Minute: Run in place, jump rope or do jumping jacks.

Do twenty seated chair dips.

1 Minute: Run in place, jump rope or do jumping jacks.

2 Minutes: Cool down by repeating stretching exercises.

The DASH Diet Cookbook

- **Chapter 11:** Breakfast

- **Chapter 12:** Lunch

- **Chapter 13:** Snacks & Appetizers

- **Chapter 14:** Dinner

- **Chapter 15:** Dessert

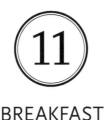

BREAKFAST

Cranberry Almond Spread

Cranberries are rich in vitamin C and almonds provide extra nutrition and crunch in this delicious fruit spread. Spoon it over yogurt for an evening dessert or spread it on a bagel for breakfast.

- 1 cup fresh cranberries
- ½ cup unsweetened orange juice
- Sugar, just a pinch
- 1 tablespoon cornstarch
- 1 tablespoon water
- ½ cup slivered almonds
- 1 teaspoon vanilla extract

Chop the cranberries then add them to a non-stick saucepan with the orange juice. Warm gently over medium heat. Add sugar to taste. Mix the cornstarch and water in a small cup until smooth. Turn the heat to low, then stir in the cornstarch mixture, raise the heat to medium-high, stir and simmer until it thickens. Remove from heat and stir in the almonds and vanilla.

Cover and chill. Store in the refrigerator up to 2 weeks.

Makes 1½ cups.

Toasted Egg Sandwich

This light breakfast provides both protein and fiber. Instead of red pepper, you may use tomato, mushroom or onion.

- Canola oil spray
- 1 slice whole wheat bread
- 2-ounce slice turkey bacon
- 1 large egg
- 1 thin slice red bell pepper, chopped
- 1 thin slice low-fat jack cheese
- Fresh-ground black pepper

Coat a non-stick skillet very lightly with canola oil spray. Over medium heat, toast the bread slice on one side in the skillet. When it's lightly browned, set aside on a plate with the toasted side of the bread facing up.

Add the turkey bacon to the skillet and cook lightly on both sides. Set this on top of the toasted bread. Break the egg into the skillet and coax it around with a spatula to about the size and shape of your slice of toast. When it's just barely set (a little softer than you like it), remove it from the skillet and set it gently on top of the open-faced sandwich.

Transfer the sandwich back into the skillet. Top it with the sliced pepper and the cheese and then cover the pan with a lid and turn the heat down to medium-low. When the cheese is melted, transfer the sandwich back to the plate and sprinkle lightly with fresh-ground black pepper to taste.

Serves 1.

Tropical Fruit and Yogurt Bowl

This combination of fruit and yogurt makes a great breakfast, but can also be served as an afternoon snack. It's loaded with vitamin C, essential enzymes and antioxidants.

- ½ cup diced fresh pineapple
- ½ cup diced fresh mango
- ½ cup diced fresh papaya
- 1 cup low-fat unsweetened yogurt
- Fresh mint
- Optional: honey, cinnamon or low-fat granola

Combine the fruit and yogurt in a bowl and stir gently. Transfer to 2 individual bowls. If desired, top each serving with a small drizzle of honey or a dash of cinnamon, or stir in a couple tablespoons of granola. Garnish with a couple fresh mint leaves.

Serves 2.

Mushroom & Swiss Omelet

Extra egg whites add protein to this easy omelet. Add olives or diced tomato if desired.

- 2 eggs plus 2 egg whites
- 1 tablespoon nonfat milk
- Canola oils spray
- ½ cup sliced fresh mushrooms
- 1 ounce low-fat Swiss cheese, cubed or shredded
- 1 small green onion, diced
- Fresh ground black pepper
- Optional: nonfat sour cream or red salsa

Warm a non-stick omelet pan on the stove over medium-low heat for about 1 minute. Meanwhile, whisk the eggs lightly with the milk. They should be just barely combined; don't over mix the eggs.

Coat the omelet pan lightly with canola oil spray and allow the pan to warm for another 15 seconds. Add the mushrooms to the pan and cook for about 1 minute, stirring once or twice.

Pour the eggs into the pan, but don't stir. When the edges begin to firm up a bit, use a heat-proof rubber spatula to slide down around the edges of the eggs and lift gently to let the liquid eggs on top flow under the edges to the bottom of the omelet pan. This works best if you lift the edges of the omelet in 4 or 5 spots around the edge of the pan.

Arrange the cheese and green onion across half of the omelet. Sprinkle with freshly ground black pepper.

Continue cooking the omelet; it will still be soft in the center. Slide a larger, flat spatula under 1 side of the omelet and fold it over the other half to form a half circle. Slide the folded omelet over a bit into the center of the pan. Use the spatula to very lightly press on the top of the omelet to coax any remaining liquid out into the pan.

Cover with a lid and remove from heat. Let the omelet sit for about 1 minute to finish setting the eggs and then slide the omelet onto a plate and serve. Top with nonfat sour cream or red salsa for extra flavor.

Serves 1.

Spring Asparagus Brunch Plate

This colorful plate provides fiber, protein and extra nutrients at breakfast or lunch. Serve it warm or chilled, with fresh fruit.

- 8 stalks young fresh asparagus
- ½ cup water
- 8 small crimini mushrooms
- 2 boiled eggs, peeled
- 1 cup plain Greek yogurt
- 1 teaspoon Dijon mustard
- 1 teaspoon honey
- 1 tablespoon fresh thyme leaves
- ¼ teaspoon turmeric
- 4 cherry tomatoes, cut into quarters
- Optional: fresh ground black pepper or nutmeg

Trim the asparagus, removing the woody bottom ends. Bring ½ cup of water to a boil in a pan large enough to hold the asparagus. Add the asparagus and mushrooms, cover with a lid and turn the heat down to medium-low.

Check the vegetables for tenderness after 5 minutes; the asparagus should be bright green but still slightly crisp. Cook another minute or 2 if necessary.

Meanwhile, chop the eggs coarsely in a microwave-safe, medium-sized mixing bowl—this is easily done using 2 knives. Add the yogurt, mustard and honey and mix lightly. Stir in the thyme and turmeric. Gently fold in the tomatoes.

Warm the egg and yogurt mixture, covered with a paper towel, in the microwave for about 45 seconds.

Use a slotted spoon to transfer the asparagus and mushrooms onto 2 plates and then spoon the warm egg and yogurt mixture over each serving. Sprinkle with fresh ground black pepper or a dash of nutmeg, if desired.

Serves 2.

Pumpkin Pie for Breakfast

This dish has the flavors of pumpkin pie without the calories. Try it for breakfast or dessert. It's healthy, easy to make and keeps for several days.

- ½ acorn squash, cut in half
- 2 apples
- 1 fresh peach
- 2 tablespoons honey
- 1 tablespoon grated fresh ginger
- ½ teaspoon cinnamon
- ¼ teaspoon nutmeg
- Ground cloves
- ½ cup low-fat peach yogurt

Remove the seeds from the squash using a spoon and cut it into large chunks. Leave the peel on, but cut the apples into quarters and remove the core. Chop the apple into bite-sized pieces. Cut the peach in half, remove the pit then cut the fruit into bite-sized pieces.

Put the squash pieces in a medium-size stockpot with about 2 inches of water. Cover and cook over medium-high heat for 10 minutes. Check the squash and add or remove water to bring the water level to about 1 inch in the pan. Add the rest of the fruit to the pan then cover and cook over medium-low heat for another 5 minutes.

Check the squash for tenderness; you should be able to easily stick a fork into it. If not, continue cooking until it's tender, making sure you maintain a bit of liquid in the pan.

When the squash is tender, use a fork or tongs to remove it from the pan to a large mixing bowl. Use a paring knife to strip off the peel. Mash the squash in the bowl and then use a slotted spoon to remove the other fruits from the pan and add them to the squash. Add the honey, ginger, cinnamon and nutmeg, along with a dash or 2 of cloves. Stir this and then cover it and chill in the refrigerator for an hour or 2. Stir in the yogurt just before serving.

Serves 2.

Strawberry Parfait Oatmeal

Oats not only provide protein, but also vitamin E, selenium, zinc, iron, copper, manganese and magnesium. Use good quality rolled oats, which are more nutritious than quick cooking or instant oats.

- ⅔ cup rolled oats
- ½ cup water
- ¼ cup nonfat milk
- ½ cup low-fat unsweetened yogurt
- ½ cup sliced strawberries
- 1 sugar-free cookie

Mix the oats, water and milk in a small saucepan and heat over medium heat. When it starts to boil, heat to low and cook for 3 minutes. Stir occasionally, with the pan uncovered, for just 3 minutes.

Remove from heat and spoon the oats into 2 parfait glasses. Top each serving with yogurt and strawberries, and then crumble the cookie over the top.

Serves 2.

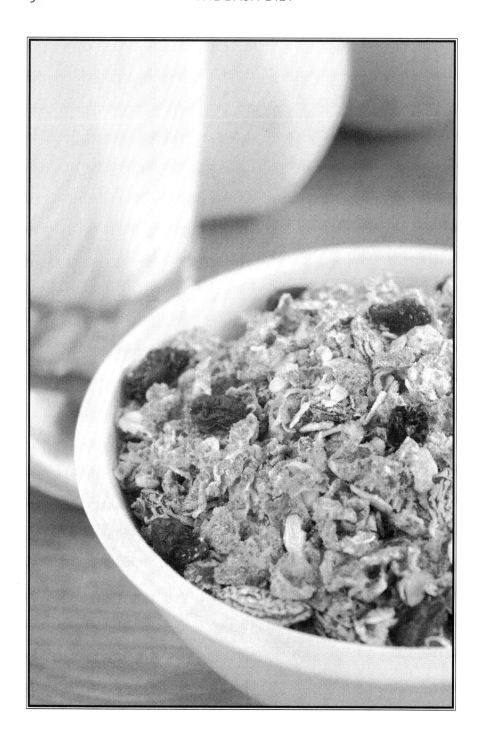

Great Grain Granola

This recipe is easy to create and makes about 12 servings. You can use also substitute rolled oats for the multi-grain mix; some commonly available mixes include oats, whole wheat, flaxseed, rye, barley and triticale.

- 4 cups multi-grain cereal mix (or oats)
- 1 cup bran cereal
- ½ cup honey
- ½ cup canola oil
- 2 apples
- Cinnamon and nutmeg
- 2 cups mixed, dried tropical fruits
- 1 cup chopped pecans

Spread the multi-grain cereal mix (or oats) and cereal mix in a large, deep, non-stick baking pan. Drizzle the honey over the top and then the oil. Stir lightly with a large spoon.

Core and quarter the apples, but don't peel them. Slice them thinly and scatter them over the multi-grain cereal mix (or oats), and then dust the top with cinnamon and nutmeg. Bake this, uncovered, in the oven at 250 degrees for about 45 minutes. Stir and toss the mixture, making sure no clumps are sticking to the bottom.

Continue baking until the oats are a golden blonde color—you do not want the mixture to be toasty brown because it will continue cooking for a little while after you take it from the oven.

Stir the mixture every 20 minutes or so until it's evenly toasted, and then remove it from the oven. Stir in the dried fruits and pecans. This is excellent served warm. When the granola is thoroughly cooled, store it in an airtight tin or a zippered freezer bag.

Serves 12.

Country Breakfast Sausage

Make your own sausage instead of eating commercially made sausage, which is often high in fat and calories. Adjust the spices to your liking.

- ½ lb. ground turkey breast
- ½ lb. lean ground pork loin
- ½ teaspoon ground sage
- ½ teaspoon minced garlic
- ½ teaspoon paprika
- ½ teaspoon black pepper
- ½ teaspoon allspice
- ¼ teaspoon onion powder
- ¼ teaspoon dry mustard

Combine all ingredients in a large bowl and mix well.

Warm a large skillet over medium-low heat and then spray it very lightly with canola oil spray. Warm the pan for another minute while forming the sausage mixture into patties of about ¾-inch thickness.

Arrange the sausage patties in the skillet and turn the heat to medium. Cook uncovered about 5 minutes on each side until well browned. Serve hot.

Optional: add cayenne or chili powder for a bit more heat. Substitute Italian seasoning herbs for the spices listed above for mild Italian sausage.

Serves 6.

Breakfast Rice Pudding

This rice pudding with nonfat milk and brown rice is healthy enough for breakfast. Double the recipe and take some to work for a snack, or save some for dessert.

- ¾ cup brown rice
- 1 tablespoon unsalted butter
- ½ teaspoon nutmeg
- ¼ teaspoon mace
- 1¼ cups water
- 1 cup nonfat milk

- 2 egg yolks
- 2 teaspoons vanilla
- 1 tablespoon sugar
- 1 teaspoon grated orange zest
- ¾ cup raisins or other dried fruit

Combine the rice, butter, nutmeg and mace in a non-stick saucepan. Toast the rice in the pan over high heat, stirring until the mixture sizzles. After about 30 seconds, add the water and stir; then cover the pan with a lid and reduce heat to very low. Do not remove the lid from the pan. Simmer the rice gently for 25 minutes and then turn off the heat and let the rice sit, covered, for another 10 minutes.

Combine the milk, egg yolks, vanilla and sugar in a blender. Blend on high for about 30 seconds and then add the orange zest (finely grated orange peel) and blend another 5 seconds.

Coat a heavy glass or ceramic baking dish very lightly with canola oil spray. Pour the milk/egg mixture into the pan and bake for 10 minutes at 350 degrees. Remove from the oven and reduce heat to 250 degrees. Stir the cooked rice gently into the warm milk, along with the dried fruit (dried cranberries or dried apricots also work really well if you don't like raisins).

Bake for 45 minutes and then stir the mixture gently, scraping the bottom of the pan. Bake another 35 minutes and check the rice—it should be semi-solid and lightly browned on top when it's done.

Serves 2.

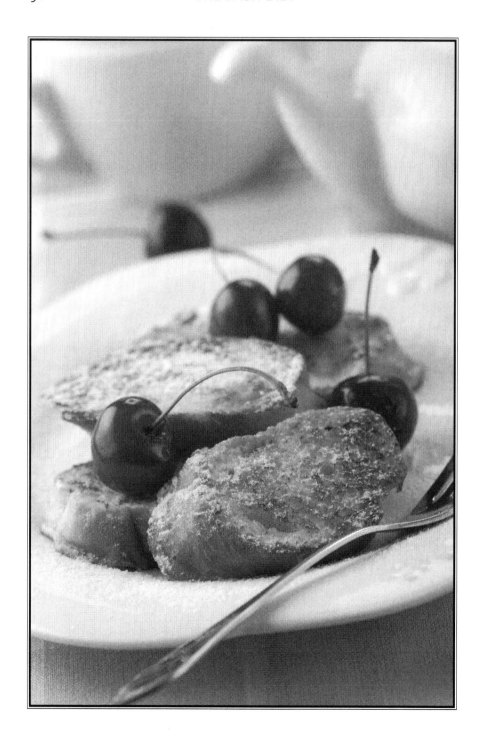

Cherry French Toast

Cherries take this breakfast standard from everyday to extraordinary. It's perfect for brunch with friends or family.

- 1 pint fresh or frozen cherries
- 1 cup water, divided
- 1 tablespoon cornstarch
- 1 tablespoon real maple syrup
- 1 teaspoon real almond extract
- 1 cup nonfat milk
- 1 egg
- ½ cup nonfat yogurt
- 3 slices whole grain bread
- Nutmeg

Combine the cherries with ½ cup water in a non-stick saucepan. Heat over medium-high heat and bring to a gentle boil. Mix the remaining ½ cup water with the cornstarch in a bowl, then stir it into the cherries. Let it simmer until thickened and remove from heat. Stir in the maple syrup and almond extract and set aside.

Preheat oven to 375 degrees.

Whisk the milk and egg together until thoroughly mixed and then whisk in the yogurt.

Lightly coat a glass baking dish with canola oil spray and then spread the cherry mixture evenly in the dish. Pour the milk mixture into a shallow pan (a pie pan works well), cut the bread slices in half and soak them in the milk mixture. Arrange them on top of the cherry mixture in the baking dish and sprinkle lightly with nutmeg.

Bake for 30–40 minutes or until the toast slices are golden brown on top. Transfer the slices with a spatula onto a plate and serve with the cherry mixture on the top.

Serves 2.

Tomato-Cheddar Omelet

Savory omelets also make a quick and easy dinner when time is short. Serve with a salad and garlic bread, fresh-sliced tomatoes, sliced black olives or fresh oranges.

- 2 eggs plus 2 egg whites
- 1 tablespoon water
- Canola oil spray
- 1 small tomato, seeded and chopped
- 1 ounce low-fat cheddar cheese, cubed or shredded
- Fresh ground black pepper
- 1 tablespoon chopped fresh cilantro

Warm a non-stick omelet pan on the stove over medium-low heat for about a minute. Meanwhile, whisk the eggs gently with the water in a mixing bowl. They should be just barely combined; don't over-mix the eggs.

Coat the omelet pan lightly with canola oil spray and allow the pan to warm for another 15 seconds. Pour the eggs into the pan, but don't stir. When the edges begin to firm up a bit, use a heat-proof rubber spatula to slide down around the edges of the eggs and lift gently to let the liquid eggs on top flow under the edges to the bottom of the omelet pan. This works best if you lift the edges of the omelet in 4 or 5 spots around the edge of the pan.

Arrange the tomato and cheese across half of the omelet. Dust with the pepper and sprinkle on the cilantro.

Keep cooking the omelet; it will still be soft in the center. Slide a larger flat spatula under 1 side of the omelet and fold it over onto the other half. Slide the folded omelet into the center of the pan. Use the spatula to very lightly press on the top of the omelet to coax any remaining liquid out into the pan.

Cover with a lid and remove from heat. Let the omelet sit for about a minute to finish setting the eggs and then slice in half and serve.

Serves 2.

Italian Toast Plate

Mediterranean style flavors provide a refreshing change for breakfast. This dish also makes a light lunch entrée. Serve with green salad.

- 1 large slice whole grain bread
- 2 teaspoons olive oil
- 2 tablespoons minced Kalamata olives
- 1 tablespoon finely diced fresh tomato
- 1 tablespoon finely diced green pepper
- 1 teaspoon minced fresh oregano
- 1 teaspoon minced fresh basil
- 1 tablespoon nonfat plain yogurt
- 1-ounce slice provolone cheese
- 1-ounce slice mozzarella cheese

Preheat the oven to 200 degrees. Brush the bread with the olive oil, place it on a plate and heat it in the oven.

Mix the olives, tomato, pepper and herbs in a bowl. Add the yogurt and stir until thoroughly combined.

Remove the toast from the oven and turn the oven heat to 375 degrees. Lay the provolone on top of the toast, and then spread the vegetable mixture over the top of the cheese. Lay the mozzarella slice on the top, and then bake on the top rack of the oven until cheese is melted and bubbly.

Serves 1.

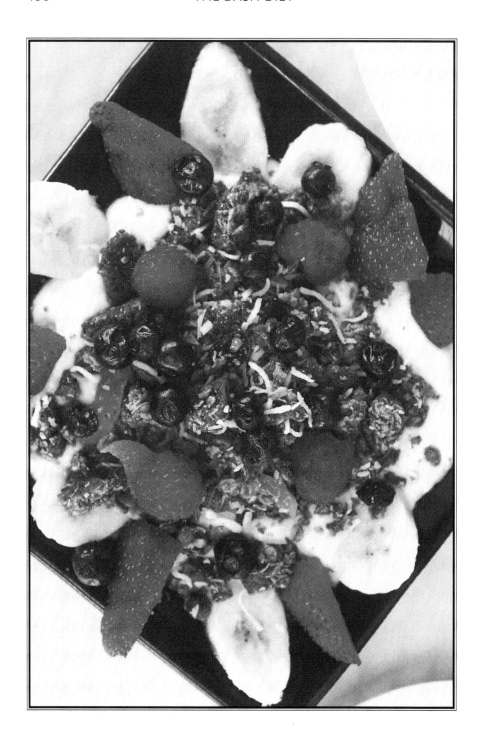

Banana-Blueberry Granola Bowl

Great Grain Granola can be used in place of store-bought granola in this recipe. On cooler mornings, heat the granola in the microwave before adding it to the yogurt.

- 1 medium banana
- ½ cup fresh blueberries
- ¾ cup nonfat yogurt
- ¼ teaspoon real almond extract
- Honey
- ¾ cup granola

Slice the banana and combine it with the berries in a mixing bowl. Stir the yogurt and almond extract together and combine this with the fruit. Drizzle lightly with honey, stir and mix with granola.

Serves 2.

Potato-Sausage Breakfast Bake

Use homemade Country Breakfast Sausage for this dish. This dish can be prepared ahead of time—just prepare and refrigerate the night before serving, then bake in the morning.

- Canola oil spray
- 1 large red potato
- 1 small sweet potato, peeled
- ½ yellow onion, peeled
- Sage and black pepper
- ½ cup unsweetened applesauce
- ¾ cup nonfat milk
- Paprika
- 2 cooked Country Breakfast Sausage patties

Lightly coat a large, glass baking dish with canola oil spray. Preheat oven to 400 degrees.

Thinly slice the potato, sweet potato and onion (about ¼ inch) and mix them together in the baking dish. Dust them lightly with the sage and black pepper.

Mix the applesauce together with the milk in a small mixing bowl and pour this over the potato mixture. Dust the top generously with paprika and set the pan on the middle rack of the oven. Bake for 30 minutes.

Cut up or crumble the cooked sausage. Remove the potato dish from the oven and gently stir the sausage into the potatoes. Add a little milk if necessary to keep the potatoes lightly coated with liquid. Bake another 20 minutes or until the potatoes are tender, browned and bubbly.

Serves 4.

Blackberry Quinoa Bowl

Native to Peru, quinoa is similar to wheat but with a subtle nutty flavor.
Serve this sweet dish warm with whole grain toast and fresh orange slices.

- ¾ cup quinoa
- 2 teaspoons canola oil
- ½ orange, peeled
- Nutmeg
- 1 cup water
- ½ cup nonfat milk
- 2 cups fresh blackberries
- 1 teaspoon vanilla

Rinse the quinoa thoroughly with cold water and drain. Heat the oil in a medium-size non-stick saucepan. Toast the quinoa in the saucepan over medium-high heat for about 1 minute, stirring constantly. Cut up the orange segments into small bite-sized pieces and remove any pits. Add a dash of nutmeg and the orange to the quinoa, stir and then add the water.

Turn the heat to low and simmer about 11 minutes, until the quinoa is almost tender but still a little crunchy in the center. Add the milk, blackberries and vanilla, stir gently and simmer another 2 or 3 minutes, until the grains of quinoa look translucent instead of opaque.

Serves 4.

Pineapple Banana Breakfast Bowl

Bananas are very low in sodium and saturated fat, and they're a good source of vitamin B6, vitamin C, potassium and manganese. Use thicker nonfat Greek yogurt for added protein.

- 1 cup nonfat yogurt
- ¼ cup unsweetened orange juice
- 1 tablespoon honey
- 1 teaspoon vanilla
- 2 large bananas
- 1 cup fresh pineapple, cut into bite-sized pieces
- ½ cup sliced seedless grapes
- ½ cup chopped, dried papaya
- 2 large pieces crystallized ginger
- Ground mace
- Optional: ½ cup shredded unsweetened coconut

Mix the yogurt, orange juice, honey and vanilla in a glass serving bowl. Cut up the bananas, pineapple, grapes and papaya and add them to the bowl. Chop the ginger very finely and sprinkle it over the fruit. Add a dash or 2 of mace on top. Stir gently and chill for at least ½ hour before serving. Add shredded coconut before serving, if desired.

Serves 4.

Bacon-Avocado Egg Dish

Avocados are low in saturated fat and sodium, but loaded with potassium, B-vitamins, vitamin E, and folic acid. Serve this open-faced sandwich with a side of yogurt or low-fat cottage cheese.

- 1 large avocado, peeled and pitted
- 2 large fresh basil leaves, thinly sliced
- 2 slices low-fat turkey bacon
- 2 eggs
- 2 large slices whole grain bread
- 2 thin slices fresh tomato
- 2 (1-ounce) slices Provolone cheese

Mash the avocado in a bowl and add the basil.

Fry the bacon in a non-stick skillet over medium heat until crispy. Drain on a paper towel.

Break the eggs into the skillet and separate them with a flat spatula. Add two tablespoons of water to the skillet, cover with a lid and turn the heat to low.

Toast the bread lightly and put a slice on each of the plates. Spread the mashed avocado over the toast, and then add the bacon strips and basil. Top with the tomato slices.

When the eggs are set, gently place 1 on each slice of toast and immediately top with sliced cheese. Cover the plates with large lids or tented sheets of foil to help melt the cheese. Serve warm.

Serves 2.

Warm Peach Granola

Use Great Grain Granola for this warm and filling breakfast bowl. It's wonderful on cooler mornings and also makes a great dessert.

- 1 large fresh peach
- ½ cup unsweetened orange juice
- ½ cup water
- ¼ cup sugar
- Cinnamon
- ¾ cup granola
- ½ cup unsweetened yogurt

Quarter and pit the peach but don't peel it. Heat the orange juice, water and sugar in a medium-size nonstick saucepan over medium-high heat until it's bubbly.

Cut the peach into bite-sized pieces and add that to the saucepan with a dash of cinnamon. Turn the heat to low and simmer 1 minute, and then add the granola. Stir gently and simmer another minute. Spoon this into a serving bowl and top with yogurt.

Serves 2.

Strawberry Pineapple Smoothie

A fruit packed smoothie provides many servings of fruit and a healthy dose of protein that'll keep you satisfied all morning. Greek yogurt has twice the amount of protein of most regular yogurts.

- 1 cup unsweetened orange juice
- ½ cup unsweetened pineapple juice
- ½ cup vanilla soy milk or low-fat vanilla soy milk
- ½ cup low-fat Greek yogurt
- ½ cup fresh strawberries
- ¼ cup pineapple chunks, rinsed and drained
- 6 ice cubes

Combine all the ingredients in a blender and blend until smooth. Pour into glasses and serve.

Serves 2.

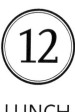

LUNCH

Southwestern Salmon

The spice mix used on the salmon can also be used on pork or chicken. Be sure to freshly grind pepper for the best flavor.

- 1 (6-ounce) salmon fillet
- 1 large Anaheim chili
- 1 medium tomato
- Canola oil spray
- Freshly ground black pepper, just a pinch
- Chili powder, just a pinch
- Cumin, just a pinch
- Onion powder, just a pinch
- ½ cup unsweetened orange juice

Rinse the salmon and pat it dry with a paper towel. Remove the stem, seeds and veins of the chili and slice it into ½-inch rings. Cut the tomato into small wedges.

Warm a non-stick skillet over medium heat and then coat it lightly with canola oil spray. Lay the salmon fillet in the middle of the skillet and then arrange the chili and tomato around it. Combine a pinch of each in a small dish: black pepper, chili powder, cumin and onion powder. Sprinkle the salmon and vegetables with the spice blend and then cover the pan with a lid.

Cook for 6 minutes and then add the orange juice. Cover the pan with the lid and turn off the heat, but leave the pan on the burner. Check the salmon for doneness after 3 more minutes. If the salmon is opaque and no longer translucent, it's done.

Serves 1.

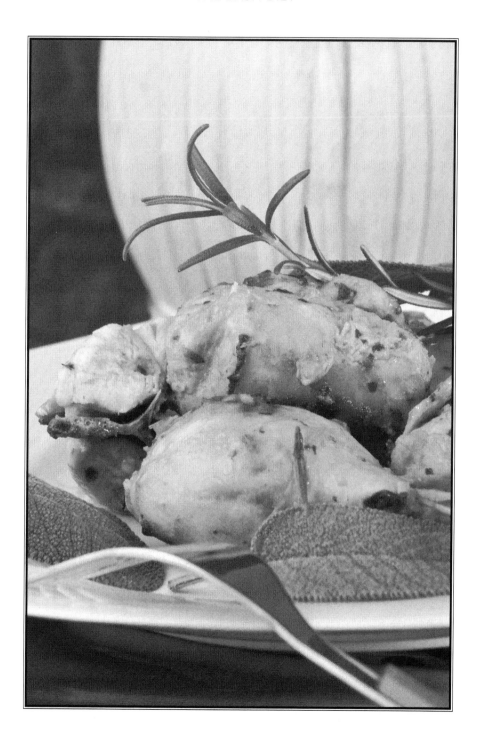

Rosemary Chicken

Quick and easy to make, this chicken dish can be served hot or cold. Try it chilled and sliced with sweet potato salad or coleslaw for lunch.

- Canola oil spray
- 1 (12-ounce) skinless chicken breast
- Black pepper
- 4 medium fresh tomatoes
- 1 tablespoon red wine vinegar
- 2 large sprigs fresh rosemary
- ½ cup dry white wine

Lightly coat an 8-inch glass baking dish with canola oil spray. Arrange the chicken in the dish and dust generously with fresh ground black pepper.

Cut the tomatoes into quarters and arrange them around the chicken. Sprinkle the vinegar over the tomatoes and then tuck the rosemary in next to the chicken. Pour the wine over into the dish, cover tightly with foil and bake for 35 minutes.

Slice the chicken breast into bite-sized pieces, toss with the rest of the ingredients and serve.

Serves 2.

Dijon Pork Chops

A lively spice blend and Dijon mustard boost flavor without any additional salt. Sautéed apples would be an excellent side dish.

- 2 boneless pork loin chops
- Canola oil spray
- ¾ cup panko breadcrumbs
- 2 tablespoons flour
- 1 teaspoon paprika
- ¼ teaspoon sage
- ¼ teaspoon garlic powder
- ¼ teaspoon chili powder
- 2 tablespoons Dijon mustard

Preheat the oven to 375 degrees. Trim the pork chops of any fat around the edge. Lightly coat a baking dish with canola oil spray.

Mix the breadcrumbs, flour and spices in a shallow bowl. Spread the mustard on 1 side of each pork chop and press that side down firmly into the breadcrumb mixture. Turn the pork chop over and press that side into the crumbs.

Set the pork chops into the baking dish with the mustard side up. Bake uncovered for 40 minutes.

Serves 2

Shrimp Kebabs

Kebabs make a tasty and attractive lunch, and they're almost fat-free. Shrimp is a good source of protein, and it's high in iron.

- 16–20 count raw shrimp (or prawns)
- ½ large fresh pineapple, peeled and top removed
- 1 red bell pepper
- 1 small red onion
- 1 tablespoon rice vinegar
- 2 tablespoons olive oil
- 1 tablespoon chopped fresh oregano
- 6 cherry tomatoes
- Cajun seasoning

Peel and devein the shrimp; drain on paper towels. Cut the pineapple into 16 chunks of about 1½ inches each.

Remove the stem and seeds from the pepper and cut it into bite-sized pieces. Cut the onion into bite-sized pieces.

Mix the vinegar, oil and oregano in a small bowl.

Thread the shrimp, pineapple, and vegetables onto skewers and lay them on a baking sheet. Brush the oil mixture over the kebabs, coating each piece well.

Preheat the grill (or prepare charcoal) and brush the kebabs again with the oil mixture. Just before grilling, dust lightly with Cajun seasoning. Grill for about 5 minutes on each side, or until the shrimp are browned on the outside and opaque on the inside.

Serves 2.

New York Turkey Melts

This recipe will help you satisfy the urge for a deli sandwich. A variety of vegetables and cheeses add to the texture and flavor of this deluxe hero.

- 4 slices low-sodium rye bread or whole wheat flatbread
- 2 tablespoons fat-free cream cheese
- 1 teaspoon prepared horseradish
- 6 ounces sliced homemade roast turkey breast
- ½ small cucumber, very thinly sliced
- ½ small red onion, very thinly sliced
- 2 thin slices provolone
- Canola oil spray

Spread 2 of the bread slices with cream cheese and horseradish and then layer on the turkey, cucumber, onion and provolone. Top each with another slice of bread.

Coat a non-stick skillet lightly with canola oil spray and toast the sandwiches over medium heat until well browned.

Serves 2.

Honey Mustard Chicken

This chicken dish is extremely quick to prepare, making it great for busy weeknights. And while you are at it, make some extra for tomorrow's lunch.

- 1 tablespoon olive oil
- 4 large skinless, boneless chicken thighs
- ½ cup slivered almonds
- ½ cup low-sodium vegetable broth
- ½ cup dry white wine
- 2 tablespoons yellow mustard
- 1 tablespoon honey
- Fresh ground black pepper

Heat a non-stick pan over medium heat, then add olive oil. Add the chicken to the pan and brown on all sides. Blend the almonds, broth, wine, mustard, and honey in a food processor until smooth. Season to taste with black pepper.

When the chicken is browned, pour the honey-mustard mixture over the chicken and cover with a lid. Turn heat to low and simmer gently for 15 minutes.

Serves 4.

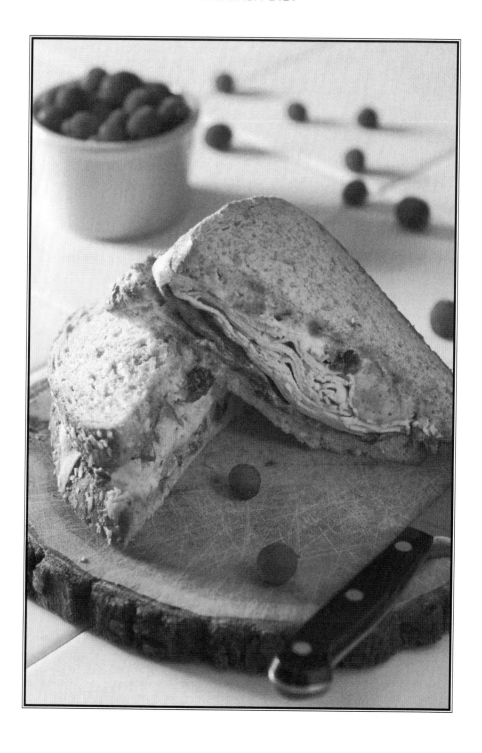

Loaded Turkey Sandwich

This recipe is great, especially when you have those Thanksgiving leftover cravings. Take it for lunch or prepare it for a quick weekend dinner.

- 1 whole wheat hoagie roll
- 1 tablespoon nonfat cream cheese
- 1 teaspoon Dijon mustard
- ½ teaspoon prepared horseradish
- 4 ounces thin-sliced homemade or low-salt deli turkey breast
- 2 tablespoons whole-berry cranberry sauce
- 1 ounce thin-sliced Swiss cheese
- 1 cup fresh alfalfa sprouts

Spread ½ of the hoagie roll with the cream cheese and the other half with the mustard and horseradish combined. Layer the turkey onto the roll with the cranberry sauce, Swiss cheese and sprouts.

Serve with a salad or cup of low-sodium soup.

Serves 1.

Lemon-Poached Cod

If you can't find cod, you can use haddock or any other firm, white fish. Serve the fish with pasta and fresh green peas.

- 2 (6-ounce) cod fillets
- Fresh ground black pepper
- 1 fresh lemon
- 1 small, fresh tomato, cut into bite sized pieces
- 4 or 5 sprigs fresh cilantro, chopped
- 1 cup water
- ½ cup white wine

Pat the cod fillets dry with a paper towel and dust them generously with black pepper. Cut half of the lemon into wedges (for serving) and then squeeze the juice from the other half into a medium-sized saucepan, large enough to hold the fish fillets.

Add the tomato and cilantro to the pan. Add the water and wine to the pan and bring to a boil over high heat. Add the cod fillets to the pan, cover tightly with a lid and remove from heat.

Let stand for 10 minutes. Serve with lemon wedges.

Serves 2.

Raspberry Spinach Salad

If raspberries aren't available, strawberries or blackberries can also be used in this elegant salad. Fresh spinach, fruit and nuts make it a nutritional powerhouse.

- 1 (6-ounce) bag baby spinach
- 1 cup fresh red raspberries
- 1 Asian pear, cut into bite-sized pieces
- ½ cup whole walnuts
- ½ cup low-fat Italian dressing
- ¼ cup low-fat blue cheese crumbles

Toss all ingredients; let stand at room temperature for 30 minutes before serving. Toss again right before plating.

Serves 2.

Grilled Chicken and Fruit Plate

An excellent warm-weather salad, the chicken can be prepared on the grill or under the broiler. For even more flavor, marinate the chicken in dressing overnight.

- 2 large, boneless, skinless chicken breasts
- Low-fat Italian dressing
- ½ cantaloupe melon
- ½ honeydew melon
- ½ fresh pineapple
- 1 cup seedless watermelon
- ½ cup unsweetened apple juice
- ½ cup low-fat mayonnaise
- Several large leaves romaine lettuce
- Pinch of ground cloves

Coat the chicken with Italian dressing then grill or broil until browned and tender. Let the chicken cool, then chill for 1 hour and slice.

Cut up the fruit into bite-sized pieces and combine in a serving bowl. Mix the apple juice and mayonnaise and stir it into the fruit mixture. Arrange the lettuce leaves on plates and top each with a quarter of the fruit salad. Sprinkle very lightly with ground cloves and then top with sliced chicken breast.

Serves 4.

Southwestern Salad

This spicy, protein-packed bean salad has plenty of tangy flavor. It is even better the next day, and makes a great potluck dish.

- 1 can black beans
- 1 can red beans
- 4 fresh tomatoes, sliced
- ½ cup chopped fresh cilantro
- 1 cup diced red peppers

- Black pepper and cumin
- 2 tablespoons olive oil
- 2 tablespoons white wine vinegar
- 1 teaspoon hot sauce

Open the cans of beans and rinse them thoroughly with cool water. Combine the beans in a serving bowl.

Add the tomatoes, cilantro and red pepper to the beans. Sprinkle generously with pepper and cumin. Whisk together the oil, vinegar and hot sauce in a small bowl and drizzle over the salad. Toss gently, cover and chill.

Let the salad stand, covered, at room temperature for 20 minutes before serving.

Serves 5.

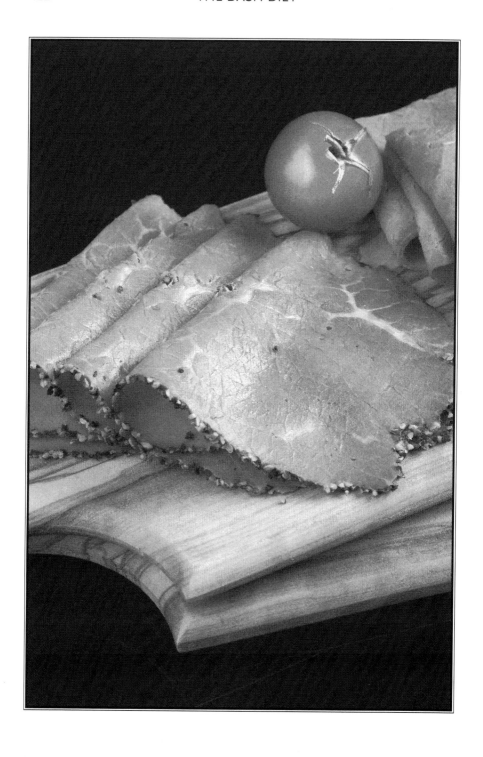

French Dip Sandwiches

Use leftover homemade roast beef rather than deli meat so you can control the sodium. Sliced roast beef can also be used in wrap sandwiches.

- 8 ounces sliced low sodium roast beef
- 1 teaspoon blackened seasoning
- 1 teaspoon canola oil
- 2 whole wheat hoagie rolls
- 1 cup black coffee
- ¼ cup water
- 2 tablespoons low-sodium Worcestershire sauce
- 1 tablespoon balsamic vinegar
- 1 tablespoon low-sodium soy sauce
- 1 tablespoon low-sodium V8 juice
- 1 tablespoon brown sugar

Preheat the oven to 300 degrees. Rub the meat with seasoning. Heat a non-stick skillet over medium-high heat. Add the oil, add the beef and brown it or thoroughly heat it.

Transfer the beef to a plate and cover with foil; wrap the hoagie rolls in foil and put the beef and the rolls in the oven to keep warm.

Add the rest of the ingredients to the skillet; stir and simmer for 3–5 minutes. Remove the beef and rolls from the oven, assemble the sandwiches and serve the au jus liquid in cups with the sandwiches.

Serves 2.

Oven-Baked Squash

This hearty side dish can also be served as a light entrée. Cooked squash can be stored in the refrigerator for up to four days and reheated in the microwave.

- 1 acorn squash
- 2 browned Country Breakfast Sausage patties
- 1 cup unsweetened applesauce
- ½ cup chopped dried apricots
- Pinch ground ginger

Cut the squash in half vertically from stem to tip. Remove the seeds and scrape away the threads of pulp.

Preheat oven to 350 degrees. Crumble the sausage into the cavities of the squash and then add the applesauce and apricots. Stir gently to combine.

Sprinkle with ginger and bake in a roasting pan or on a rimmed cookie sheet for 1 hour, or until tender.

Serves 2.

Fresh Broccoli Salad

This salad is best served at room temperature. You can add sliced seedless grapes, or use raisins instead of the cranberries if you prefer.

- 1 large bunch broccoli
- 2 strips turkey bacon, fried crisp and chopped
- 1 cup chopped fresh spinach
- ½ cup dried cranberries
- 2 small carrots, shredded
- ½ small red onion, diced fine
- ½ cup low-fat mayonnaise
- ¼ cup low-fat French dressing
- 1 tablespoon honey

Chop the head of the broccoli into small florets and shred the long stems coarsely using a box grater or food processor. Combine both stems and florets in a serving bowl with the bacon, spinach, cranberries, carrots and onion.

Whisk together the mayonnaise, dressing and honey together in a small mixing bowl and pour this over the salad. Toss and serve.

Serves 5.

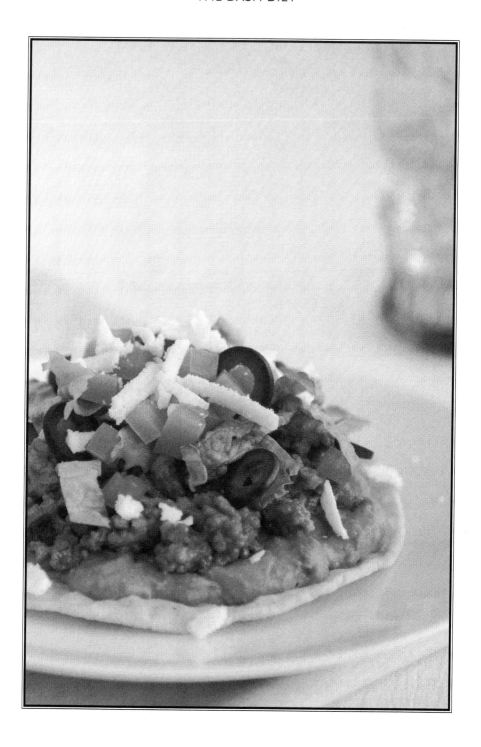

Beef Tostadas

These colorful tostadas are a one dish meal and healthier than fast food Mexican food. You can use ground turkey breast instead of beef if you prefer.

- ½ pound extra-lean ground beef
- Black pepper, just a pinch
- Chili powder, just a pinch
- Cumin, just a pinch
- 1 (16-ounce) can nonfat refried beans
- ½ cup low-sodium V8 juice
- 4 crispy tostada shells
- 2 cups shredded low-fat Swiss cheese
- 2 cups shredded lettuce
- 2 cups chopped fresh tomato
- ¾ cup diced white onion
- ¾ cup sliced black olives

Heat a skillet over medium heat. Brown the ground beef in the skillet, crumbling with a wooden spoon. Season the beef with cumin, black pepper and chili powder to taste. When thoroughly cooked, add the beans and the juice and stir. Reduce the heat to low and keep warm.

Set the tostada shells on plates and top each with a serving of the beef/bean mixture. Top each tostada with shredded cheese and then the lettuce, tomato, onion and olives.

Serves 4.

Arroz con Pollo

Rice and chicken is a delicious and nutritious traditional Latin American dish. You can turn the leftovers into a hearty soup by combining with chicken broth.

- ¼ cup canola oil
- ¾ pound boneless, skinless chicken breast, cut into bite-sized pieces
- Black pepper, turmeric and cumin
- ½ cup chopped yellow onion
- ½ cup chopped celery
- 1 teaspoon minced garlic
- 2 cups low-sodium chicken broth
- 1 cup white basmati rice
- ½ cup chopped cilantro
- 2 Serrano peppers, diced fine

Heat a large stockpot over medium heat and add the oil. Toss the chicken with the spices and add to the pot. Cook the chicken then add the onion, celery and garlic and continue cooking, stirring until the chicken is browned on all sides.

Add the chicken broth and turn heat to high. When the mixture boils, add the rice, cilantro and peppers. Cover with a lid and turn the heat to very low. Simmer another 15 minutes. Serve hot with warm tortillas and fresh tomatoes.

Serves 4.

Summer Sweet Potato Salad

This riff on traditional potato salad has loads of flavor, color and texture. It's a more nutritious alternative to potato salad made with red or white potatoes.

- 4 large sweet potatoes
- 1 large white onion, chopped
- 2 boiled eggs, peeled and chopped
- 2 green onions, chopped
- 4 radishes, sliced
- ½ cup chopped celery
- ½ cup low-fat mayonnaise
- ½ cup nonfat sour cream
- 2 tablespoons yellow mustard
- 1 tablespoon chopped fresh dill
- Fresh ground black pepper

Fill a saucepan with water and place on the stove. Cut the potatoes into bite-sized pieces and add to the saucepan. Bring the pan to a boil over medium heat and boil the potatoes until just barely tender. Drain and chill for 1 hour.

In a large serving bowl, combine the potatoes, onion, eggs, green onions, radishes and celery. Mix together the mayonnaise, sour cream, mustard and dill. Stir this into the potato mixture and season with black pepper. Chill for an hour before serving.

Serves 4.

Asian Cod Lunch

If cod is not available, substitute another firm white fish such as halibut or haddock. The bright Asian flavors add tang and accent the freshness of the fish.

- Orange juice
- 2 tablespoons olive oil
- 2 tablespoons dry mustard
- 1 tablespoon honey
- 1 tablespoon rice vinegar
- 2 teaspoons grated fresh ginger
- 2 teaspoons low-sodium soy sauce
- 3 tablespoons unsweetened orange juice
- 2 (6-ounce) cod fillets
- Canola oil spray
- ½ cup sliced green onions
- ½ cup diced fresh tomato

Mix the orange juice, oil, mustard, honey, vinegar, ginger and soy sauce together in a non-reactive glass or plastic (not metal) bowl. Add the cod fillets and marinate in the refrigerator, covered, for 45 minutes.

Lightly coat a non-stick skillet with canola oil spray and heat over medium heat. Add the fillets and then nestle the green onions and tomato around the fillets in the pan. Cook for 1 minute.

Gently turn the fish over with a wide spatula and add the rest of the marinade. Cover with a lid and turn the heat to low. Cook for 2 minutes. Serve the cod on top of steamed rice, with the vegetables and sauce over the top.

Serves 2.

Artichoke Chicken

This dish is creamy and decadent, but guilt-free. Serve with whole wheat pasta or a crusty whole wheat roll.

- Canola oil spray
- 2 boneless, skinless chicken breasts
- 1 can artichoke hearts (not marinated)
- 1 can diced tomatoes
- ½ cup frozen spinach, drained
- ½ cup dry white wine
- 2 slices Provolone cheese
- Salt substitute, to taste

Preheat oven to 375 degrees. Lightly coat a baking pan with canola oil spray. Arrange the chicken in the pan.

Drain and rinse the artichoke hearts and add them to the chicken. Add the tomatoes and spinach, then pour the wine into the pan.

Cover and bake 30 minutes. Uncover the dish, lay the cheese on top and bake for 5 more minutes. Season to taste with salt substitute.

Serves 2.

Avocado Halibut

This fish dish has a bit of a kick, so beware of the heat. Serve with sliced fresh tomatoes and a green salad.

- Canola oil spray
- 2 (6-ounce) halibut fillets
- 2 ripe avocados, peeled and pitted
- ½ cup mild green salsa
- ½ cup nonfat Greek yogurt
- 1 fresh jalapeño, seeded and diced

Preheat the broiler. Lightly coat a broiler pan with canola oil spray. Set the fillets on the pan. Mash the avocados and mix in the salsa, yogurt and *jalapeño*. Warm this mixture in a non-stick saucepan over low heat.

Place the halibut fillets on the broiler pan and broil for 5 minutes and then turn them over and broil another 4 minutes. Serve the halibut with the warmed guacamole sauce on top.

Serves 2.

(13)

SNACKS & APPETIZERS

Garlic-Basil Shrimp

You can make these on skewers if you'd like. Just soak the skewers in water for 30 minutes to prevent them from burning, then cook as directed.

- 1 tablespoon unsalted butter, melted
- 16–20 count raw shrimp (or prawns)
- 12 large fresh basil leaves
- 2 tablespoons minced garlic
- ½ cup dry white wine

Preheat the broiler and add the butter to a broiler-safe pan. Peel and devein the shrimp and then wrap each one as tightly as possible with a basil leaf. Add the garlic and spread it evenly around the pan and then add the wrapped shrimp. Broil for 1 minute and then turn the shrimp over and add the wine. Broil again until the shrimp are done, about 4 minutes.

Serves 2.

Stuffed Mushrooms

Parmesan cheese is high in sodium, so save these for special occasions. You can also substitute low-fat shredded mozzarella to reduce the sodium.

- 12 large fresh mushrooms
- ¼ cup grated Parmesan cheese
- ½ cup panko breadcrumbs
- 2 tablespoons finely chopped green onion
- ¼ cup nonfat sour cream

Preheat the broiler. Remove the stems from the mushrooms and chop the stems very finely. In a bowl, combine the mushrooms, cheese, breadcrumbs and green onion.

Stir in the sour cream and mix well. Stuff the caps of the mushrooms with the mixture. Place the mushrooms on a broiler pan and broil until mushrooms are tender and browned.

Serves 4 as an appetizer or 2 as a light lunch.

Watermelon Smoothie

This smoothie makes a refreshing snack or dessert. Freeze the ingredients and blend to create a fruity sorbet.

- 4 ice cubes
- 1 tablespoon unsweetened orange juice
- 3 cups seedless watermelon, cut into small chunks
- 1 cup strawberries, stems removed
- Optional: fresh mint

Pulse the ice and orange juice in a blender until the ice is broken up and then add the watermelon and berries. Blend until smooth; garnish with a fresh mint leaf if desired.

Serves 2.

Avocado Cheese Melts

Mashed avocado is sometimes a good substitute for butter. It adds richness to this twist on a grilled cheese sandwich.

- 1 ripe avocado, peeled and pitted
- 4 slices whole grain bread
- 4 ounces thin-sliced Swiss cheese

Mash half of the avocado in a bowl and slice the other half thinly. Spread the mashed avocado on the bread slices and top each with a slice of cheese. Arrange the sliced avocado on top of the cheese. Broil for several minutes, until the cheese is melted.

Serves 4.

Shredded Carrot Salad

Carrots and cranberries provide vitamin C and vitamin A. Serve this as a side dish or on a chicken sandwich.

- 1 large carrot, shredded
- ½ cup low-fat yogurt
- 1 tablespoon dried cranberries
- Cinnamon and mace
- Optional: 1 tablespoon crushed pineapple

Combine the carrot, yogurt and cranberries in a bowl. Add a dash of cinnamon and mace and stir. Add a spoonful of crushed pineapple, if desired.

Serves 1.

Italian Tomato Salad

This salad has the flavors of bruschetta or an Italian antipasto platter. Serve with some crusty bread to sop up the dressing.

- 1 cup cherry tomato halves
- ½ cup black olives, rinsed and drained
- 1 small Anaheim chili, sliced
- ¼ cup diced red onion
- 1 tablespoon chopped fresh basil
- 1 tablespoon chopped fresh oregano
- 1 teaspoon chopped fresh rosemary
- 1 tablespoon balsamic vinegar
- 1 teaspoon honey
- 1 tablespoon olive oil
- ½ cup fresh low-fat mozzarella cheese, cubed

In a bowl, combine the cherry tomatoes, olives, chili, onion and herbs. Sprinkle the vinegar over the salad and drizzle on the honey and olive oil. Fold in the mozzarella. Serve at room temperature.

Serves 2.

Chicken Quesadilla

These quesadillas are comforting and filled with protein. Serve with a side of guacamole or nonfat sour cream.

- 2 small flour tortillas
- 1 tablespoon green salsa
- ½ cup shredded, cooked chicken
- ½ cup low-fat shredded cheddar cheese
- Chili powder, just a pinch
- Cumin, just a pinch

Preheat the broiler. Set one of the tortillas on a baking sheet and spread the salsa over the top of it. Arrange the chicken on top and then add half of the cheese. Sprinkle with cumin and chili powder. Lay the second tortilla on top and press it down firmly onto the chicken mixture.

Sprinkle with the remaining cheese, place on a broiler pan and broil until the cheese is melted. Cut into wedges and serve.

Serves 2.

Pineapple Smoothie

This smoothie is loaded with protein, healthy fats, and fruits, but it'll remind you of a tropical cocktail. It's also delicious frozen.

- 1 cup unsweetened pineapple juice
- ½ cup unsweetened orange juice
- 1 cup vanilla soy milk or low-fat vanilla soy milk
- ½ cup low-fat Greek yogurt
- ½ cup pineapple chunks, rinsed and drained
- 1 teaspoon vanilla
- 6 ice cubes

Combine all the ingredients in a blender and blend until smooth. Pour into 2 glasses and serve.

Serves 2.

Chewy Granola Bars

These nutritious and fiber-rich snack bars are easy to make. Stash them in your desk for snacking.

- Canola oil spray
- 2 cups uncooked 5-grain cereal
- 1 cup chopped, dried tropical fruit
- ½ cup bran flakes
- ½ cup toasted wheat germ
- ½ cup chopped walnuts
- ½ cup dry nonfat milk powder
- ¾ cup honey
- ¾ cup unsalted peanut butter
- 1 tablespoon canola oil
- 1 tablespoon vanilla

Preheat oven to 325 degrees. Lightly coat a 9 x 13-inch baking pan with canola oil spray. Combine the cereal, dried fruit, bran flakes, wheat germ, walnuts and dry milk in a mixing bowl. Whisk together the honey, peanut butter and canola oil in a non-stick saucepan and heat over medium heat.

Don't let the mixture boil; when it's hot, remove from heat and add the vanilla. Pour the warm mixture over the dry ingredients and stir quickly until well mixed.

Spread the mixture evenly into the baking pan and flatten it with a large metal spatula so it's firmly set in the pan. Bake for 20 minutes.

Set the pan on a rack to cool for 15 minutes and then cut into 24 snack-size bars. Remove from the pan. Store in an airtight tin with waxed paper between layers, or wrap each one in foil. Store for up to 1 week.

Serves 24.

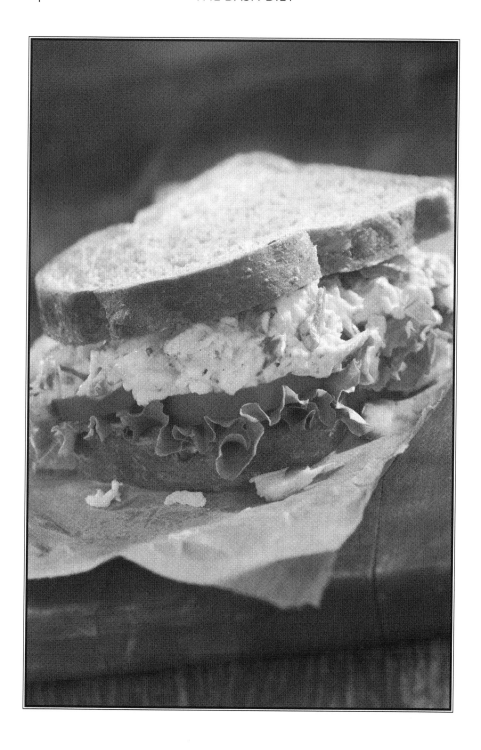

Summer Chicken Salad

This chicken salad is a great warm-weather entrée and an excellent way to use leftover chicken. Wonderful on its own, you can also use it as a sandwich or pita bread filling.

- 3 cups cooked, skinless chicken breast
- ½ cup chopped celery
- ½ cup chopped apple
- ¼ cup chopped almonds
- ¼ cup low-fat mayonnaise
- 2 teaspoons chopped fresh sage
- 2 teaspoons chopped fresh cilantro

Combine all the ingredients in a bowl and stir until combined. Chill for an hour before serving.

Serves 6.

Sugar-Free Applesauce Cookies

A terrific snack or dessert for work or picnics, these cookies keep very well in a tightly closed container, or you can freeze them for up to a month.

- 1 cup rolled oats
- ½ cup unbleached flour
- ½ cup whole wheat flour
- 2 teaspoons cinnamon
- 1 teaspoon baking soda
- 1 teaspoon nutmeg
- ½ teaspoon cloves
- 1 cup unsweetened applesauce
- 1 cup raisins
- ½ cup canola oil
- ½ cup chopped pecans
- 2 eggs
- 2 teaspoons vanilla
- Canola oil spray

Preheat oven to 375 degrees. Mix the oats, flours, spices, and soda in a large mixing bowl. Combine the remaining ingredients in another bowl and mix thoroughly. Combine the wet and dry ingredients.

Coat a baking sheet with canola oil spray. Drop by spoonful onto the baking sheet, leaving space between each cookie. Bake for 8 or 9 minutes. Do not over bake.

Makes 4 dozen.

Zesty Fresh Salsa

Serve this delicious salsa with fat-free tortilla chips. It's a great party dish to make ahead.

- 4 Roma tomatoes
- 2 ripe tomatillos, peeled of their papery skin
- 1 small red onion
- 2 Serrano chilies
- ½ cup chopped fresh cilantro
- 1 tablespoon chopped fresh oregano
- 2 teaspoons minced garlic
- 1 teaspoon cumin
- 3 fresh limes
- Fresh ground black pepper
- Optional: hot sauce

Chop the tomatoes, tomatillos, onion and Serrano chilies very finely and combine in a bowl. Stir in the cilantro, oregano, garlic and cumin. Grate the peel of 1 lime very finely and add the peel to the mix.

Juice the limes and add the juice. Season to taste with black pepper. Add hot sauce to taste.

Serves about 4.

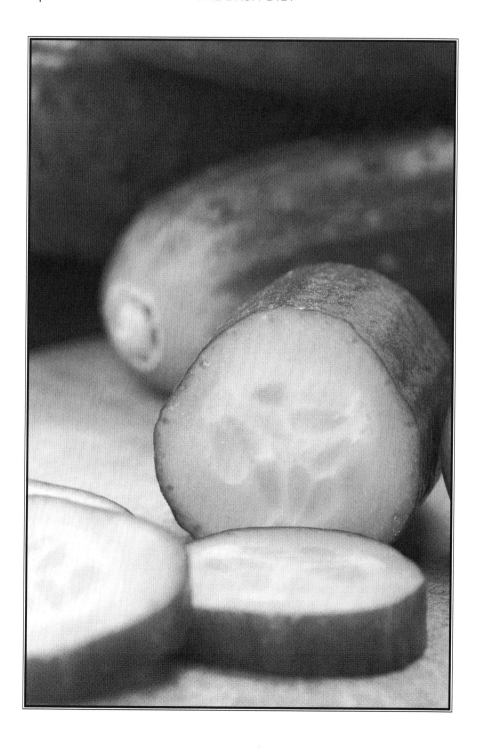

Zesty Cucumber Salad

This makes a good side dish served with fish or seafood. It can also be served as a very refreshing light snack.

- 1 medium cucumber, sliced very thin
- ½ fresh red grapefruit, chopped
- ¼ cup rice vinegar
- ¼ cup sesame oil
- ½ teaspoon sugar
- 1 tablespoon black or white sesame seeds

Mix the cucumber and grapefruit together in a bowl. Stir the vinegar, oil and sugar together in a cup and then pour over the cucumbers. Sprinkle with sesame seeds and serve chilled.

Serves 2.

Creamy Salmon Dip

Serve this with crackers or a plate of carrots, celery, jicama and radishes for dipping. Fresh dill can be used in place of the dill pickle relish if desired.

- 1 (6-ounce) steamed salmon fillet
- 1 cup nonfat Greek yogurt
- ½ cup finely diced red onion
- 1 teaspoon dill pickle relish
- 1 teaspoon horseradish
- Nutmeg
- Fresh ground black pepper

In a mixing bowl, break up the salmon with a fork and stir in the yogurt, onion, relish and horseradish. Add a dash of nutmeg and then season to taste with black pepper.

Serves 4.

Crisp Pear Salad

This salad features the Mediterranean flavors of walnuts, feta and grapes. It tastes even better the next day, so prepare the night before you plan on serving it.

- 2 cups fresh romaine leaves, torn
- 1 Asian pear, cored and chopped
- ½ cup feta cheese, crumbled
- ¼ cup walnuts, chopped
- 8 seedless grapes, sliced in half
- 1 tablespoon chopped fresh mint
- 1 tablespoon fresh lemon juice
- 2 tablespoons olive oil

Toss together the lettuce, pear, feta, walnuts, grapes and mint. Dress the salad with lemon juice and olive oil and toss again. Serve chilled.

Serves 2.

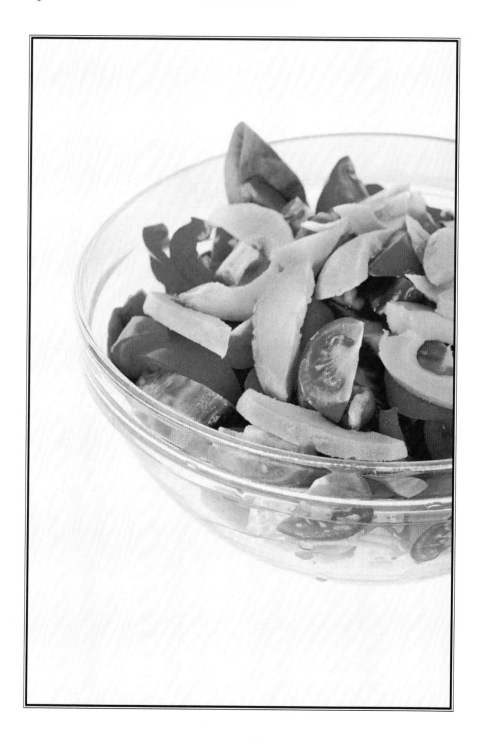

Zesty Avocado Salad

The fresh flavors of this salad are perfect for a summer picnic. For a spicier version, leave the pepper seeds in or add ½ cup green salsa.

- 1 large ripe avocado, peeled and pitted
- 4 cherry tomatoes, halved
- ½ cup chopped fresh cilantro
- 2 jalapeños, seeded and chopped
- ½ cup diced red onion
- ½ fresh orange, peeled and chopped
- 1 teaspoon minced garlic
- 2 fresh lemons
- 2 tablespoons olive oil

Cut the avocado into bite-sized pieces. Combine in a serving bowl with the tomatoes, cilantro, jalapeños, onion, orange and garlic.

Grate the peel of 1 lemon very finely and add the peel to the bowl. Juice both of the lemons and add the juice to the bowl. Drizzle with olive oil and serve.

Serves 2.

Creamy Seafood Salad

This salad is great on its own or as a sandwich filling. Serve with low-sodium crackers or a bowl of soup.

- 6 ounces fresh cooked crab or low-sodium artificial crab
- 4 ounces fresh cooked bay shrimp
- 2 green onions, diced
- ½ cup finely chopped celery
- ½ cup finely chopped fresh grapefruit
- ¼ cup low-sodium Italian salad dressing
- ¼ cup fat-free sour cream
- ¼ teaspoon ground cardamom
- 1 teaspoon chopped fresh cilantro
- Head of romaine

Combine all ingredients with the exception of the romaine in a salad bowl and chill. Serve on a bed of romaine lettuce.

Serves 4.

Crunchy Apple Salad

This healthier version of the classic Waldorf salad is vegetarian, but still packed with protein. Serve with sandwiches or a cup of soup.

- 2 large apples, cored and cut into small, bite-sized chunks
- ½ cup chopped celery
- ½ cup chopped pecans
- ½ cup sliced seedless grapes
- ½ cup unsalted peanut butter, or tahini
- ½ cup nonfat yogurt
- Cinnamon and nutmeg

Combine the apples, celery, pecans and grapes in a bowl. Whisk together the peanut butter and yogurt and add to the salad. Stir to combine. Garnish with a couple dashes each of cinnamon and nutmeg.

Serves 2.

Sweet Potato Almond Bread

Sweet potatoes make this quick bread wonderfully moist. Store for up to one week. Great toasted for breakfast.

- Canola oil spray
- 1 medium sweet potato, peeled and boiled
- 1 small banana
- ½ cup nonfat milk
- ¾ cup brown sugar
- 2 eggs
- ¾ cup chopped almonds
- 1 tablespoon canola oil
- 1 teaspoon nutmeg
- ½ teaspoon cinnamon
- ½ teaspoon ginger
- 1 cup whole wheat flour
- ½ cup unbleached flour
- ½ cup crushed bran flakes cereal
- 1 teaspoon baking powder
- 1 teaspoon baking soda

Preheat oven to 350 degrees and coat a loaf pan with canola oil spray. Dust it lightly with flour.

Mash the sweet potato and banana together and then add the milk. Mix well. Blend in the sugar and the eggs. Mix in the almonds, oil and spices. Combine the dry ingredients and add them to the sweet potato mixture.

Pour the batter into the loaf pan and smooth the top. Bake for 35 minutes and test for doneness. Cool on a rack for 10 minutes before removing from pan.

Serves 8.

Minted Snow Pea Salad

This lighter version of a classic layered salad is great for lunch or as a side dish served with fish or shellfish. If you like, you can add a bit of fresh tarragon.

- 2 cups fresh or frozen snow peas, cooked and chilled
- 2 boiled eggs, peeled
- ½ cup nonfat sour cream
- 1 tablespoon olive oil
- 1 tablespoon chopped fresh mint
- Fresh ground black pepper

Put the peas in a glass serving bowl. Chop the eggs fine and mix with the sour cream and olive oil. Stir in the mint and add to the peas. Stir lightly and season with black pepper.

Serves 2.

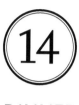

DINNER

Tender Lemon Chicken

Light and mild lemon chicken is good hot or cold. Double or triple this recipe and you'll have a key ingredient to make salads or sandwiches for lunch the next day.

- 2 (6-ounce) boneless, skinless chicken breasts
- Fresh ground black pepper
- 2 long sprigs fresh thyme
- 1 (12-ounce) can sugar-free lemonade

Preheat oven to 350 degrees. Arrange the chicken in a non-stick baking dish. Season generously with pepper and then top each piece of chicken with a sprig of thyme. Pour the lemonade in the dish.

Cover tightly with foil and bake for 30 minutes. Serve with rice and fresh peas or sweet corn.

Serves 2.

Italian Beef Stew

You can substitute ground turkey or chicken breast in this hearty stew to make it even leaner. This recipe can be made in a slow cooker: Brown the beef then cook with the other ingredients on low for 6–8 hours.

- ½ pound extra-lean ground beef
- 1 small yellow onion, chopped
- 1 cup sliced fresh mushrooms
- 1 tablespoon minced garlic
- 1 tablespoon Italian seasoning
- 1 cup tomato juice
- 1 cup black coffee
- ¾ cup dry red wine
- 1 cup orzo

Brown the beef with the onion in a large non-stick stockpot over medium heat. Add the mushrooms, garlic, Italian seasoning and stir occasionally for 2 or 3 minutes. Add the tomato juice, coffee, and wine. When the liquid begins to simmer, add the orzo.

Stir gently, cover with a lid and simmer on low heat for 15 minutes.

Serves 6.

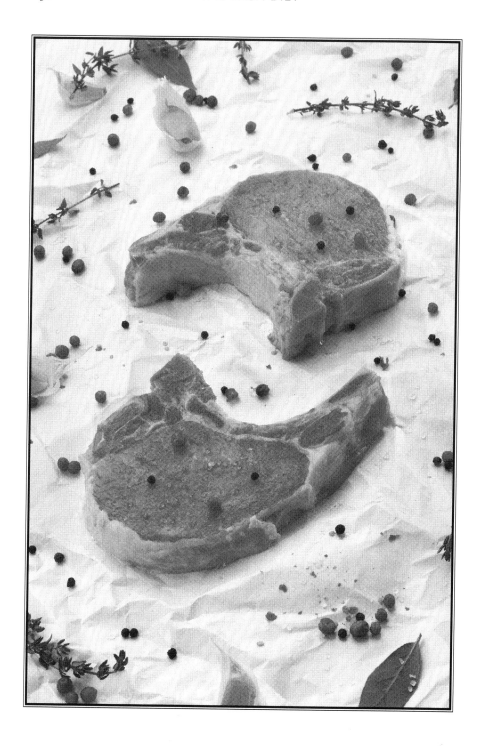

Pork Chops With Garlic Sweet Potatoes

Garlic sweet potatoes are a wonderful accompaniment to pork. If you have fresh herbs on hand, add a few snips of rosemary, thyme or tarragon.

- 2 large sweet potatoes
- 1 tablespoon minced garlic
- Sage and black pepper
- 2 boneless lean pork chops
- Dry mustard
- 1 cup nonfat milk

Slice the potatoes into ½-inch slices and toss them in a bowl with the garlic. Season lightly with ground sage and black pepper. Spread the potatoes in a non-stick baking pan and top with the pork chops.

Dust the pork chops lightly with dry mustard and then pour the milk into the pan and onto the potatoes.

Cover and bake at 375 degrees for 30 minutes then uncover and bake for another 10 minutes.

Serves 2.

Broccoli-Rice Bake

Add leftover chicken or turkey to this side dish and turn it into a quick and easy entrée. Frozen vegetables will get soggy, so they're not suitable for this dish.

- 3 cups chopped fresh broccoli
- 1 cup chopped fresh cauliflower
- ½ cup finely chopped carrots
- ½ cup sliced fresh mushrooms
- ¾ cup long grain and wild rice blend
- ½ cup shredded low-fat Swiss cheese
- 1 cup nonfat milk
- 1 cup nonfat sour cream

Combine the vegetables in a bowl and toss together. Add the rice and cheese. Mix the milk and sour cream together and pour it over the broccoli mix.

Cover and bake at 375 degrees for 45 minutes, or until rice is tender.

Serves 6.

Spicy Southwest Chili

This hearty chili definitely delivers on flavor, and the leftovers are even better the next day. For a leaner version, use ground turkey or chicken.

- ½ pound extra-lean ground beef
- 1 cup chopped yellow onion
- 2 cans red beans, rinsed and drained
- 1 can black beans, rinsed and drained
- 1 (12-ounce) can low-sodium V8 juice
- ½ cup chopped celery
- 1 tablespoon minced garlic
- 4 Roma tomatoes, chopped
- 2 Anaheim chilies, seeded and chopped
- 2 Serrano chilies, seeded and chopped
- 1 tablespoon low-sodium chili powder
- 2 teaspoons cumin
- 1 teaspoon oregano

Brown the ground beef in a large non-stick stockpot. Add the remaining ingredients and stir. Simmer over very low heat for at least an hour.

Serves 6.

Pork Loin With Apricots

This elegant and sophisticated dish is perfect for a dinner party. Serve with brown rice and fresh green beans.

- 1 pound pork tenderloin
- 1 (8-ounce) package dried apricots
- 1 cup water
- 1 cup cooking sherry or dry white wine
- 1 teaspoon chopped fresh sage
- 1 teaspoon chopped fresh rosemary
- Fresh ground black pepper and paprika

Set the tenderloin in a non-stick baking dish and tuck the apricots all around. Add the water and wine and sprinkle the herbs over the apricots. Season the pork generously with pepper and paprika. Cover with foil and bake at 375 degrees for 45–50 minutes.

Serves 4–5 people.

Easy Chicken Burritos

Use leftover chicken to make this delicious Southwestern entrée. Serve with fresh salsa and a dollop of guacamole.

- ½ pound shredded, cooked, skinless chicken breast
- 1 can fat-free refried beans
- 1 cup low-fat shredded jack cheese
- 1 cup finely chopped fresh spinach
- 1 cup chopped fresh tomatoes
- ½ cup shredded lettuce
- ½ cup sliced black olives
- 4 large flour tortillas
- ½ cup nonfat sour cream or plain nonfat yogurt

Combine the chicken and the beans in a non-stick saucepan over medium heat. In a large bowl, combine the cheese, spinach, tomatoes, lettuce and olives.

Warm the tortillas in a non-stick skillet over low heat and then spread each 1 with ¼ of the chicken/bean mixture and ¼ cup of cheese.

Top with a handful of the vegetable mixture and a spoonful of sour cream, then fold up tightly into burritos.

Serves 4.

Mushroom Turkey Cutlets

Herbs pair well with turkey, so feel free to substitute tarragon or sage instead of cilantro and oregano. Leftovers can be used for making hot open-faced sandwiches.

- 1 tablespoon canola oil
- 4 (4-ounce) turkey breast cutlets
- 2 cups sliced fresh mushrooms
- 1 cup low-sodium chicken broth
- ½ cup dry white wine
- 1 tablespoon cornstarch
- 1 tablespoon chopped fresh cilantro
- 1 tablespoon fresh oregano

Heat a large non-stick skillet over medium heat. Add the oil and brown the turkey. When browned well on all sides, add the mushrooms and chicken broth. Turn heat to medium-high.

Combine the wine and cornstarch in a small bowl, then stir that into the simmering broth. Add the cilantro and oregano and simmer over very low heat for 15 minutes before serving.

Serves 4.

Honey-Mustard Pork Chops

These freeze very well, so double the recipe if you like. Serve with a fresh green vegetable and brown rice or sweet potatoes.

- Canola oil spray
- ½ cup panko breadcrumbs
- 1 tablespoon cornstarch
- 1 teaspoon paprika
- 1 teaspoon chili powder
- 2 tablespoons Dijon mustard
- 1 tablespoon honey
- 2 boneless lean pork chops

Preheat oven to 375 degrees. Lightly coat a baking dish with canola spray. Mix the breadcrumbs, cornstarch, paprika and chili powder together in a shallow bowl.

Mix the mustard and honey together in another bowl. Dip the pork chops into the honey-mustard mixture and then into the breadcrumb mixture.

Set the pork chops in the baking dish and bake uncovered for 35 minutes.

Serves 2.

Chicken & Lentil Bake

This rustic French style dish of chicken and lentils is pure comfort. Serve with a green salad and a crusty whole wheat baguette or rolls.

- 4 boneless, skinless chicken thighs
- 1 cup finely chopped carrots
- 1 cup green lentils
- ½ cup chopped onions
- ½ cup chopped fresh sage
- 1 cup nonfat milk
- ½ cup cooking sherry or dry white wine
- ½ cup low-sodium chicken broth
- Nutmeg and black pepper

Preheat oven to 350 degrees. Arrange the chicken in a deep non-stick baking dish. In the pan add the carrots, lentils and onions. Sprinkle with sage.

Combine the milk, sherry and broth in a small bowl and pour over the dish. Add a couple dashes of nutmeg and a generous pinch of black pepper.

Bake uncovered for 45 minutes, or until lentils are tender.

Serves 4.

Beef & Mushroom Stew

This beef stew has lots of ingredients but takes little effort to prepare and can be made in a slow cooker. After browning the beef, add all of the ingredients to the slow cooker and cook on low heat for 6–8 hours.

- 1 tablespoon canola oil
- 1 teaspoon minced garlic
- ¾ pound lean stew beef, cut into chunks
- 1 tablespoon apple cider vinegar
- 1 tablespoon low-sodium Worcestershire sauce
- 1 teaspoon brown sugar
- 2 teaspoons hot sauce
- Black pepper
- ½ cup dry red wine
- 1 cup low-sodium V8 juice
- 1 cup low-sodium vegetable broth
- 2 cups small whole mushrooms
- 3 small sweet potatoes, cut into bite-sized pieces
- 1 large carrot, cut into bite-sized pieces
- 1 cup cut-up fresh green beans
- 1 can no-salt diced tomatoes

Heat the oil and garlic in a skillet over medium-high heat. Add the beef and sauté until browned on all sides. Add the vinegar, Worcestershire, sugar and hot sauce and then season generously with black pepper. Pour in the wine, V8 juice and broth. Reduce heat to a simmer and add the vegetables. Simmer on low until the vegetables are tender. Serve over whole wheat pasta or brown rice.

Serves 4.

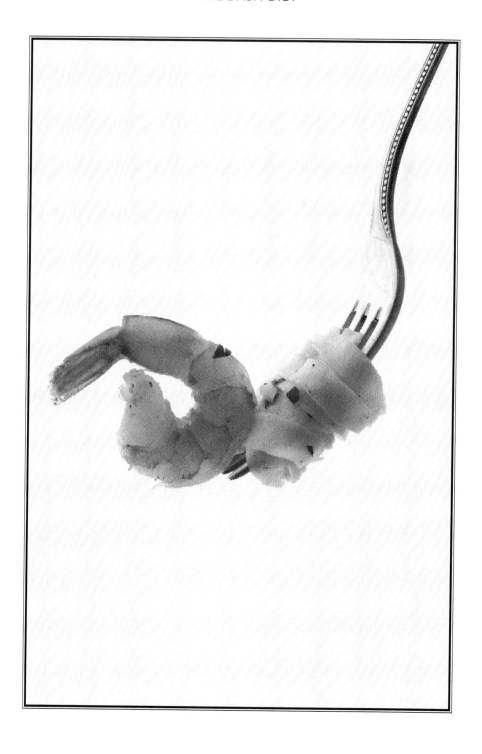

Seafood Fettuccine

Pasta is delicious and nutritious when topped with fresh vegetables, herbs and seafood instead of rich sauces and cheese. If you prefer, you can substitute low-sodium artificial crab for the shrimp and crab.

- 10 ounces dry fettuccine noodles
- 3 tablespoons minced garlic
- 1 tablespoon olive oil
- 2 medium tomatoes, cut into bite-sized pieces
- 1 green bell pepper, cut into bite-sized pieces
- 2 tablespoons chopped fresh basil
- 2 tablespoons chopped fresh oregano
- ½ pound cooked bay shrimp
- ½ pound cooked crab

Boil the fettuccine per package directions. Meanwhile, combine the garlic and oil in a large non-stick skillet and heat gently over medium heat. Add the tomatoes and peppers to the skillet.

Stir in the basil and oregano, add the shrimp and crab and cook just until the seafood is heated. Drain the pasta and stir it into the skillet.

Serves 4.

Artichoke Shrimp & Scallops

This is a festive seafood dish that will please guests. For an appetizer, serve warm with crostini. As a main dish, serve over rice or pasta with a green salad.

- ¼ pound cooked peeled shrimp
- ¼ pound cooked bay scallops
- 1 (14-ounce) can artichoke hearts, drained and rinsed
- 1 tomato, chopped
- 1 cup low-sodium spicy V8 juice
- ½ cup lemon juice
- 1 tablespoon chopped fresh cilantro

Combine all ingredients in a large saucepan and cook over medium heat just until the seafood is heated.

Serves 2.

Easy Spaghetti Squash

Spaghetti squash can be used as a substitute for pasta, but it's also great as a vegetable side dish. Baking brings out its nutty flavor beautifully.

- 1 medium spaghetti squash
- 2 slices turkey bacon, fried crisp and crumbled
- 2 Roma tomatoes, chopped
- 1 small bell pepper, chopped
- 1 teaspoon caraway seeds

Preheat oven to 350 degrees. Cut the squash vertically from stem to tip. Bake cut-side up for 45 minutes, or until tender. Remove squash from oven and scrape the insides into a large glass baking dish.

Fluff squash with a fork until the fibers are separated then add the bacon, tomatoes, pepper and caraway. Toss lightly and return to oven for another 10 minutes before serving.

Serves 2.

Ham and Pineapple Bake

*This ham dish has plenty of fruit and vegetables, and sweet tropical flair.
Serve with a green vegetable and salad.*

- Canola oil spray
- ¾ pound lean, low-sodium turkey ham
- 3 fresh yams or sweet potatoes
- 1 fresh pineapple
- 1 cup unsweetened orange juice or pineapple juice
- 1 red bell pepper

Lightly coat a baking dish with canola oil spray. Cut the ham into 2-inch chunks.

Peel the yams and cut them into 1-inch pieces. Cut the pineapple into bite-sized pieces. Combine the ham, yams and pineapple in the baking dish; add the juice and enough water to reach 1 inch deep in the pan.

Cover and bake at 350 degrees for 45 minutes. Chop the pepper finely and add that to the baking dish; bake 5 more minutes before serving.

Serves 4.

Hawaiian Chicken

The tropical flavors add brightness to this chicken dish. Fresh pineapple is best, but you can use drained chunks of canned pineapple in a pinch.

- 6 (6-ounce) boneless, skinless chicken breasts
- Paprika and black pepper
- ½ pineapple, peeled and cubed
- ½ cup rice vinegar
- ¼ cup golden raisins
- 1 small chopped white onion
- 1 orange chopped bell pepper
- ¼ cup brown sugar
- 1 tablespoon minced fresh ginger
- ½ teaspoon cinnamon
- 1 teaspoon turmeric
- 1 tablespoon cornstarch

Season the chicken breasts with paprika and black pepper and grill or broil them until cooked through, or until internal temperature reaches 165 degrees.

Combine the pineapple, vinegar, raisins, onion, pepper, brown sugar, ginger, turmeric and cinnamon in a large saucepan and cook over medium heat.

Blend the cornstarch with ½ cup water and add to the hot mixture; stir and simmer for 5 minutes and then spoon the mixture over chicken breasts before serving.

Serves 6.

Spicy Sausage & Bean Stew

Portuguese home style cooking inspires this stew. It's a hearty meal especially satisfying on cold nights.

- 2 tablespoons olive oil
- ½ cup chopped onion
- ½ pound Italian chicken sausage, crumbled
- 2 cans garbanzo beans
- 1 can diced tomatoes
- 2 cups low-sodium chicken broth, divided
- 1 teaspoon chopped oregano
- 1 teaspoon fennel seed

Cook the onions with the oil over medium heat in a heavy stockpot for about 3 minutes. Add the sausage and cook for 4 minutes or until browned.

Drain and rinse 1 can of garbanzo beans and add to the sausage and onion.

Combine the other can of beans with the tomatoes and 1 cup of broth in a blender; blend until almost smooth and pour this into the pan, and then add the rest of the broth with the oregano and fennel.

Simmer uncovered for 30 minutes.

Serves 4.

Thai Chopped Chicken Salad

This delicious Asian salad is bright and tangy. Enjoy it as a salad, or use it to fill a whole wheat wrap.

- ¾ pound cooked chicken breast
- ¾ cup cooked brown rice
- ¾ cup fresh lime juice
- ½ cup chopped cilantro
- ½ cup unsalted, roasted cashews
- 2 green chopped onions
- 1 small chopped cucumber
- 1 small can crushed pineapple, drained, or fresh pineapple
- ¼ cup chopped fresh mint
- ¼ cup diced red onion
- ¼ cup olive oil
- ¼ teaspoon cayenne pepper
- 1 head chopped romaine lettuce

Combine all the ingredients except the cayenne and romaine in a large serving bowl. Toss to combine.

Sprinkle with cayenne, then toss with the romaine and chill for 30 minutes before serving.

Serves 4.

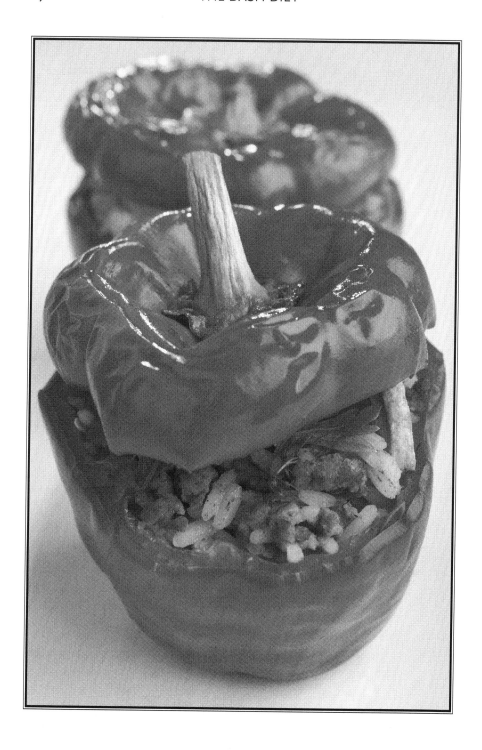

Southwestern Stuffed Peppers

If you'd like, you can substitute ground turkey breast for the ground beef. Red peppers are preferred, but you can also use orange or yellow.

- 4 large red bell peppers
- ½ pound extra lean ground beef, cooked
- 4 cups cooked brown rice
- ½ cup chopped onions
- ½ cup chopped tomatoes
- 1 Serrano chili, diced
- 1 cup nonfat sour cream
- Cinnamon and cayenne
- Cumin and chili powder

Cut the peppers in half vertically from stem to tip and remove the seeds and ribs.

In a large bowl, combine the ground beef, rice, onions, tomatoes, Serrano chili and sour cream. Add a dash or 2 of cinnamon and cayenne and then season generously with cumin and chili powder.

Stuff each half of the bell peppers with the beef/rice mixture and arrange them in a baking dish.

Add just enough water to reach ½ inch in the pan, and then bake at 400 degrees for 30 minutes. Check the peppers; if they're not yet tender, then bake another 15 minutes.

Serves 4.

DESSERT

Banana Cream Yogurt

Enjoy the flavors of banana cream pie without all the fat. This is a great dessert to give the kids.

- 1 medium banana
- 1 graham cracker
- 1 teaspoon fresh lemon juice
- 1 cup nonfat vanilla yogurt

Slice the banana into a bowl. Break the graham cracker into small pieces and add to the banana. Sprinkle with lemon juice and top with yogurt.

Serves 1.

Baked Coconut Custard

This dessert is a bit high in saturated fat, so enjoy it as an occasional treat to serve company. For a chocolate version, add a tablespoon of cocoa before blending and baking.

- Canola oil spray
- 2 cups nonfat milk
- 1 cup unsweetened flaked coconut
- 4 eggs
- ¾ cup sugar
- ¼ cup melted unsalted butter
- 1 tablespoon vanilla
- 2 dashes nutmeg
- Optional: sugar-free gingersnap cookies

Coat a nonstick 10-inch pie pan with canola oil spray. Combine all ingredients in a blender and blend 1 minute.

Pour into pie pan and bake at 350 for 45 minutes, or until custard is set. If desired, top with a couple crushed cookies.

Serves 4.

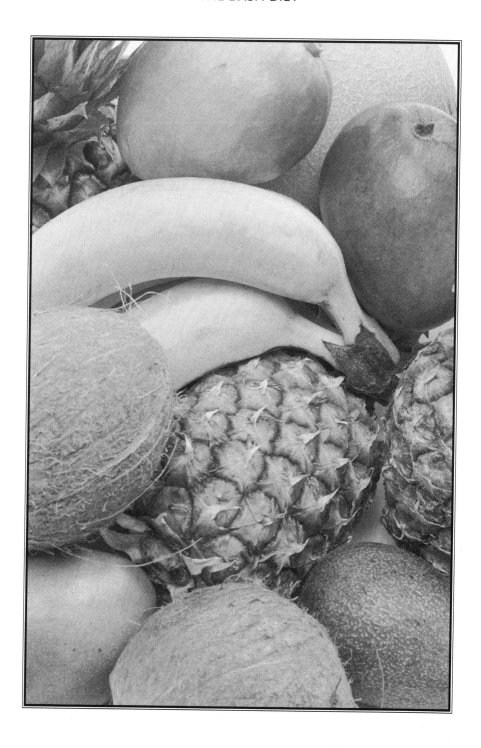

Tropical Fruit Bowl

This tropical fruit salad can be served for breakfast or dessert. It can be made a day before serving.

- 1 cup fresh pineapple chunks
- ½ cup chopped orange
- ½ cup chopped, dried papaya
- 1 banana, sliced
- ½ cup unsweetened, flaked coconut
- 1 cup low-fat yogurt
- 1 medium piece crystallized ginger, finely chopped
- 1 teaspoon vanilla
- Dash of nutmeg

Combine all the fruit and the coconut. Mix the yogurt, ginger and vanilla together and stir into the fruit. Top with a dash of nutmeg.

Serves 4.

Easy Meringue Cookies

These freeze very well if wrapped or sealed tightly. If you want to transport them, freeze them first, as they'll be less likely to crumble.

- 3 egg whites
- ½ teaspoon cream of tartar
- ⅓ cup sugar
- 1 teaspoon vanilla
- 1 cup unsweetened shredded coconut
- 1 cup sugar-free chocolate chips
- ½ cup chopped almonds

Preheat oven to 400 degrees. Beat the egg whites until frothy. Add the cream of tartar and continue beating until the meringue stands in peaks. Add the sugar gradually. Add the vanilla. With a large rubber spatula, carefully fold in the coconut, chocolate chips and almonds.

Line a cookie sheet with a silicone baking mat or parchment. Drop the mixture by spoonful onto the pan, forming cookies about the size of a large strawberry.

Put the pan in the hot oven, turn the heat off and leave the door shut. Do not remove the cookies until the oven is cold and the cookies are completely cool.

Makes 12.

Strawberry Blintzes

Frozen crepes are the basis for this easy dessert or breakfast dish. If you prefer, fill the crepes with any other berries instead of strawberries.

- 3 frozen crepes
- 1 cup nonfat ricotta cheese
- 6 fresh strawberries

- 2 teaspoons vanilla
- ¾ cup sugar-free orange marmalade

Thaw the crepes in the refrigerator and then heat them in the microwave for 30 seconds under a damp paper towel. Lay the crepes on plates, add the ricotta and sliced berries, and then roll up into a packet like a burrito. Mix the vanilla and marmalade and spoon it over the tops of the crepes.

Serves 3.

Pear Bars

These moist bars will keep for up to a week, so be sure to wrap them well. Take them to work for a morning or afternoon snack or pack them in school lunch boxes.

- 2 cups crushed sugar-free cookies
- ½ cup unsalted butter, melted
- 2 eggs
- ½ cup brown sugar
- 1 teaspoon vanilla
- ⅓ cup flour
- ½ teaspoon ground ginger
- ¼ teaspoon baking powder
- 2 medium pears, cored and diced
- ½ cup unsweetened, flaked coconut
- ½ cup chopped dried apricots

Preheat oven to 350 degrees. In a small mixing bowl, combine crushed cookies and melted butter. Press into a lightly greased 9-inch square glass pan. Bake 20 minutes.

Beat the eggs, sugar and vanilla. In a separate bowl combine flour, ginger and baking powder. Stir into egg mixture and then fold in the pears, coconut and apricots. Spread this mixture over the warm crust. Bake another 20 minutes, or until nicely browned. Cool on a rack and cut these into bars while still slightly warm.

Makes 1 dozen.

Coffee Cup Chocolate Cake

An individual cake is good when you are craving a chocolate treat. Be sure your mug is microwave safe.

- 4 tablespoons sugar
- 4 tablespoons flour
- 2 tablespoons cocoa
- 1 tablespoon cornstarch
- 2 tablespoons egg, whisked
- 1 tablespoon sugar-free strawberry jam
- 3 tablespoons nonfat milk
- 3 tablespoons canola oil
- 3 tablespoons sugar-free chocolate chips
- ½ teaspoon vanilla

Mix the dry ingredients with a fork in a large coffee mug and then add the egg and jam and mix well.

Add the milk and oil and mix thoroughly. Stir in the chocolate chips and vanilla.

Microwave on high for 2–3 minutes (depending on power of microwave). Let cool for 1 minute before serving.

Serves 1.

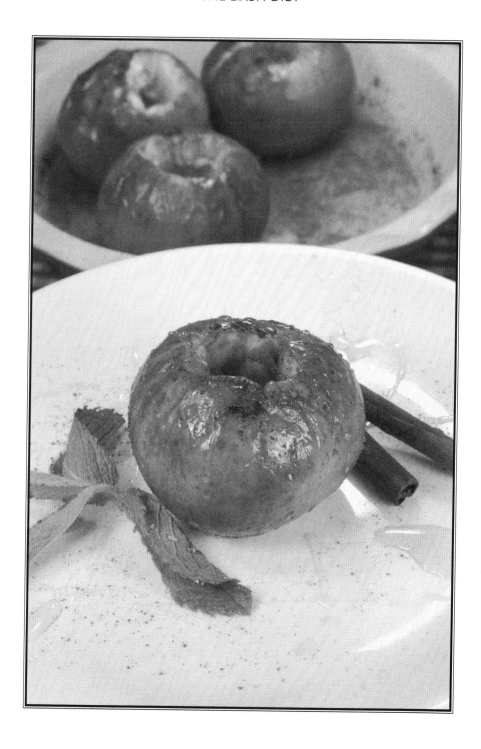

Baked Cinnamon Apples

This might be the perfect autumn dessert to serve with low-fat cheese or ice cream. If you don't care for dates, use the more traditional filling of raisins or currants.

- ¼ cup finely chopped pecans
- ¼ cup finely chopped dates
- Juice and grated peel of 1 orange
- ½ teaspoon cinnamon
- 4 apples
- 1 cup unsweetened apple juice
- 1 cup unsweetened orange juice
- 3 tablespoons brown sugar
- 2 tablespoons cold water
- 1 tablespoon cornstarch

Preheat oven to 350 degrees. Mix the pecans, dates, orange and cinnamon. Remove the cores from the apples, working from the top, but leave about ½ inch at the bottom of the apple so it's not completely hollow. Spoon the pecan and date filling into the cored apples.

Set the stuffed apples into an 8-inch square baking dish. Pour in the juices and cover the dish with foil. Bake for 30 minutes and then remove the apples to 4 dessert plates.

Pour the juices from the baking pan into a medium-sized saucepan. Simmer the liquid over medium-low heat for 5 minutes and then add the sugar. Whisk together the cold water and cornstarch in a small bowl and pour it into the simmering juice. Stir until it thickens. Serve the sauce spooned over the baked apples.

Serves 4.

Chocolate Mocha Mousse

Elegant enough for company but quick enough for a weeknight treat. For a fancier presentation, freeze the mousse in sundae glasses or pretty teacups.

- 1 (12-ounce) package sugar-free chocolate chips
- ½ cup sugar
- 1 cup boiling black coffee
- 3 eggs
- 1 teaspoon vanilla

Combine the chocolate chips and sugar in the blender. Turn the blender on high and slowly pour in the boiling coffee. Keep the blender running and add the eggs, 1 at a time. Turn the blender to low, add the vanilla and blend another 10 seconds.

Pour the mixture into 8-ounce glasses and set them in the freezer. You can eat this frozen, or just leave it in the freezer until it sets. Serve chilled.

Serves 4.

Apricot Sorbet

Use the most delicious and ripe apricots for this summer dessert. If you don't have good fresh apricots, use firm peaches or nectarines instead.

- 4 fresh apricots
- ¼ cup unsweetened orange juice
- 2 tablespoons sugar
- 1 teaspoon almond extract
- Ground ginger and mace

Combine apricots, juice, sugar and almond extract in a food processor. Blend on high until the mixture is smooth. Add a dash each of ginger and mace and blend another 5 seconds.

Spoon into 2 bowls and freeze until slushy; stir well and freeze another 30 minutes before serving.

Serves 2.

Guilt-Free Gingersnap Cookies

These spicy cookies are packed with flavor but have almost no fat at all. If you want them to keep and stay moist, store them in an airtight container with a slice of bread.

- 3 eggs
- 2 cups brown sugar
- ½ teaspoon baking powder
- ½ teaspoon baking soda
- 2 teaspoons cinnamon
- 2 teaspoons ginger
- ½ teaspoon cloves
- ¼ teaspoon nutmeg
- 2 cups flour

Preheat oven to 350 degrees. Combine the ingredients in order, beginning with the eggs and ending with the flour; drop small spoonsful onto a well-greased cookie sheet. Bake 8 or 9 minutes, or until firm.

Makes 2 dozen.

Pineapple Bread Pudding

This tropical pudding is a huge hit with kids. Serve cold, at room temperature, or warm with a dollop of plain or vanilla yogurt.

- Canola oil spray
- 6 slices whole wheat bread
- 1 cup fresh pineapple chunks
- ½ cup chopped dates
- Cinnamon and nutmeg

- 3 eggs
- 1 cup nonfat milk
- 1 cup unsweetened yogurt
- ½ cup brown sugar

Preheat oven to 375 degrees. Lightly coat an 8-inch glass baking pan with canola oil spray. Cut the bread into small cubes and transfer them to the pan. Arrange the pineapple and dates evenly over the bread and sprinkle with cinnamon and nutmeg.

Combine the eggs, milk, yogurt and sugar in the blender and blend for about 30 seconds. Pour this over the bread and press the mixture down gently with a flat spatula to compress the bread a bit. Sprinkle the top with just a little brown sugar.

Bake for 30 minutes, or until golden brown.

Serves 4.

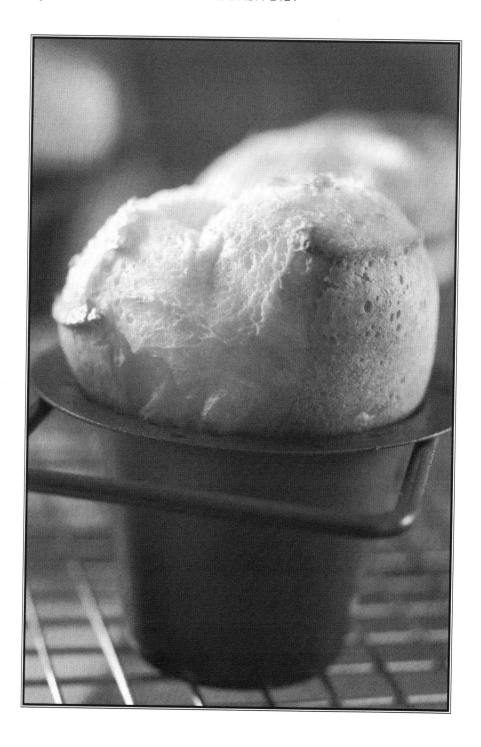

Golden Popovers

Traditionally served with roasts, popovers are a wonderful accompaniment to soup or salad, or even dessert. Serve popovers warm with fruit preserves, or at room temperature with nonfat vanilla pudding or ice cream.

- Canola oil spray
- 1 cup nonfat milk, at room temperature
- 1 cup flour
- 2 eggs
- 1 tablespoon canola oil
- ¼ teaspoon salt

Preheat oven to 400 degrees and set the oven rack to the lower third level. Coat the cups of a muffin pan with canola oil spray.

Combine the milk, flour, eggs, oil and salt in a food processor; blend for about 30 seconds. Scrape down the sides of the processor and blend another 15 seconds.

Pour the batter into the muffin cups until they are just a little more than half full. Bake until the popovers are puffed and golden brown, about 35 minutes. Do not open the oven door while baking or the popovers will collapse. Serve warm or allow them to cool to room temperature.

Makes 8.

Rhubarb Crunch

Rosy rhubarb is loaded with antioxidants and vitamin C. This sweet and sour dessert with soft fruit and crunchy topping freezes well.

- 6 cups chopped rhubarb
- ¾ cup sugar
- 3 tablespoons flour
- Canola oil spray
- ¾ cup brown sugar
- ¾ cup rolled oats
- ¾ cup flour
- ½ cup chopped walnuts
- ¼ cup unsalted butter
- ¼ cup canola oil

Preheat oven to at 375 degrees. Combine the rhubarb, sugar and flour in a large bowl. Coat a 9 x 13-inch glass baking dish with canola oil spray. Transfer the rhubarb mixture to the pan.

To make the topping combine the brown sugar, oats, flour, walnuts, butter and oil in a mixing bowl. Crumble the topping over the rhubarb and spread evenly.

Bake for 35 minutes. Serve warm with sugar-free ice cream, or serve chilled.

Serves 8.

Rich Applesauce Cake

A surprising combination of ingredients is the basis of this extremely moist cake. It can be frozen and is great served with coffee.

- 2 cups sugar
- 2½ cups flour
- 1 teaspoon baking soda
- ¾ teaspoon cinnamon
- ½ teaspoon allspice
- ½ teaspoon cloves
- ¼ teaspoon baking powder
- 1 cup raisins

- ½ cup unsalted soft butter
- ½ cup chopped walnuts
- ½ cup coffee
- 1½ cups unsweetened applesauce
- ¾ cup fat-free mayonnaise
- Canola oil spray

Preheat oven to 350 degrees. Mix first 7 ingredients together well, using a stand mixer on low speed. Add raisins, butter, walnuts and coffee. Mix on medium speed for another 2 minutes. Add the applesauce and mayonnaise and beat 2 more minutes. Spray a 9 x 13-inch pan with canola oil spray, spread the cake batter evenly in the pan and bake for 45–50 minutes or until a toothpick inserted into the center of the cake comes out clean. Allow the cake to cool on a wire rack before cutting into squares and serving.

Serves 12.

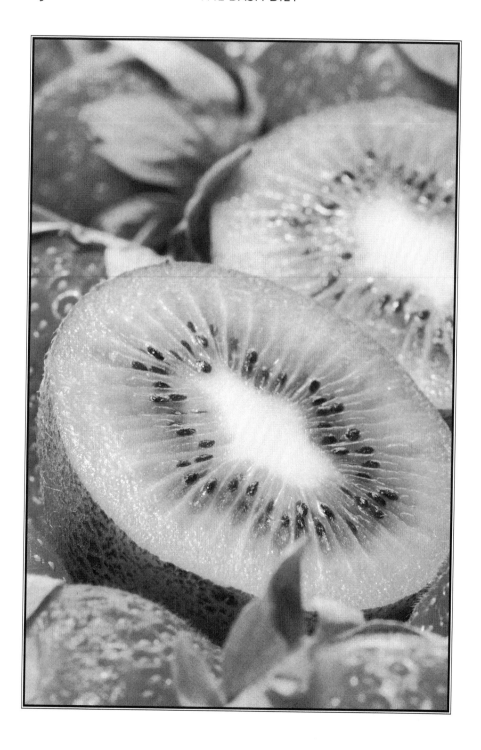

Strawberry Kiwi Smoothie

This smoothie makes a vitamin C packed breakfast, snack or dessert. For variety, use blackberries or raspberries instead of strawberries.

- 1 cup fresh strawberries
- 2 kiwi fruits, peeled and cut into quarters
- 1 cup unsweetened yogurt
- 1 cup nonfat milk

Add strawberries, kiwi, yogurt and milk to the blender. Blend on high until smooth.

Serves 2.

Hot Fudge Mocha Cake

The traditional favorite chocolate cake has been modified for DASH. The unconventional technique yields a rich chocolate cake with hot fudge sauce on the bottom of the pan.

- 1 cup flour
- 1 cup sugar
- ¼ cup cocoa
- 2 teaspoons baking powder
- ½ cup nonfat milk

- ¼ cup canola oil
- 1 teaspoon vanilla
- 1 cup brown sugar
- 3 tablespoons cocoa
- 1¾ cups hot coffee

Preheat oven to 350 degrees. Mix first 4 ingredients in a bowl. Stir in the milk, oil and vanilla, and spread the batter into a greased 9-inch square pan.

Mix the cocoa and brown sugar in a bowl, and spread this over the chocolate batter, then pour the hot coffee slowly over the top of the mixture. Do not stir. Bake for 40 minutes.

Serves 6.

Chocolate Mint Drop Cookies

These treats may remind you of a certain Girl Scout cookie. Crispy at first, these meringue style cookies become chewy over time. Store in an airtight container for up to three days.

- 3 egg whites
- ½ teaspoon cream of tartar
- ⅓ cup sugar
- 1 teaspoon mint extract
- 1 cup sugar-free white chocolate chips

Preheat oven to 400 degrees. Beat the egg whites until frothy. Add the cream of tartar and continue beating until the meringue stands in peaks. Add the sugar gradually and then the extract. With a large rubber spatula, gently fold in the chocolate chips.

Line a cookie sheet with a silicone baking mat or baking parchment. Drop the mixture by spoonful onto the pan, forming cookies about the size of a large strawberry.

Put the pan in the hot oven, turn the heat off, and leave the door shut. Do not remove the cookies until the oven is completely cold.

Makes 1 dozen.

Microwave Custard

This easy pudding is rich and creamy, yet relatively low in fat. Almond, hazelnut or maple extract in place of vanilla will give it a whole new flavor.

- 1 cup nonfat milk
- 2 eggs
- 2 tablespoons sugar
- 1 tablespoon fat-free cream cheese
- 1 tablespoon grated lemon peel
- 1 teaspoon vanilla
- Pinch of nutmeg

Heat milk in a saucepan over medium-low heat until it's almost boiling.

Meanwhile, combine the remaining ingredients in a blender and blend until smooth. When the milk is almost boiling, turn the blender on high and very slowly pour the milk into the blender.

Pour the mixture into 6 lightly greased 6-ounce custard cups. Set them in the microwave, uncovered, on a tray.

Microwave for 5 minutes and then check to see if the custard is set. If not, microwave another minute or 2, until the custard is set firmly. Serve warm or chilled.

Serves 6.

Berry Banana Smoothie

This smoothie works for dessert, a cool snack or even a fast breakfast. Store fruit in the freezer to whip up cool smoothies in a hurry.

- 1 banana, cut into 4 pieces
- 1 cup fresh or frozen blueberries
- 1 cup unsweetened yogurt
- 1 cup nonfat milk
- 1 teaspoon almond extract

Add banana, blueberries, yogurt, milk and almond extract to the blender. Blend on high until smooth.

Serves 2.

CONCLUSION

The DASH diet and DASH to Fitness Plan are a roadmap towards a healthier lifestyle.

The flexibility of the diet and exercise program is designed to enable you to make necessary changes as easily as possible. As your health and fitness improves, modify the program to fit your personal needs.

Backed by scientific research, the DASH diet is not a quick fix—it's a new way of living and a commitment to better health.

Endorsed by the National Institutes of Health, and backed by several health organizations such as the Mayo Clinic and the American Heart Association, the DASH diet's methods are built on sound nutritional advice:

- **Reduce sodium** to lower hypertension or the risk of hypertension.
- **Increase fiber** to reduce blood pressure, steady blood sugar levels and aid in weight loss.
- **Minimize saturated fat and trans fat** to increase heart health, lower LDL (bad) cholesterol, raise HDL (good) cholesterol, aid in weight loss and decrease risk/symptoms of heart disease, diabetes and metabolic syndrome.
- **Increase intake of healthy fats** by eating nuts, seeds, fish, avocado and other Omega-3 rich foods.

The recipes in *The DASH Diet Health Plan* are just the beginning. The next steps are yours to take. We wish you health and success on your DASH diet journey.

APPENDIX

Endnotes

1 "Guide to Lowering High Blood Pressure," National Heart, Lung and Blood Institute http://www.nhlbi.nih.gov/hbp/prevent/h_eating/h_eating.htm.

2 "DASH Diet: Healthy Eating to Lower Your Blood Pressure," MayoClinic.com, 15 May, 2010, http://www.mayoclinic.com/health/dash-diet/HI00047.

3 "US News & World Reports: Best and Healthiest Diet Plan," Dashdiet .org, http://dashdiet.org/.

4 "Managing High Blood Pressure with a Heart-Healthy Diet," American Heart Association, 4 April, 2012, http://www .heart.org/HEARTORG/Conditions/HighBloodPressure/PreventionTreatmentofHighBloodPressure/Managing-Blood-Pressure-with-a-Heart-Healthy-Diet_UCM_301879_Article.jsp.

Bibliography

Appel, Lawrence J; Moore, Thomas J; Obarzanek, Eva; Vollmer, William; Svetkey, Laura; Sacks, Frank; Bray, George; Vogt, Thomas et al. "A Clinical Trial of the Effects of Dietary Patterns on Blood Pressure." The New England Journal of Medicine (Massachusetts Medical Society) 335 (1997): 1117–1124. DOI:10.1056/NEJM199704173361601. ISSN 0028-4793. PMID 9099655.

Blumenthal, James A., PhD; Babyak, Michael A., PhD; Hinderliter, Alan, MD; Watkins, Lana L., PhD; Craighead, Linda, PhD; Lin, Pao-Hwa, PhD; Caccia, Carla, RD; Johnson, Julie, PA-C; Waugh, Robert, MD; Sherwood, Andrew, PhD. "Effects of the DASH Diet Alone and in Combination With Exercise and Weight Loss on Blood Pressure and Cardiovascular Biomarkers in Men and Women With High Blood Pressure." Arch Intern Med. 170(2) (2010): 126–135. doi:10.1001/archinternmed.2009.470. http://archinte.jamanetwork.com/article.aspx?articleid=415515.

Chobanian, Aram; Bakris, George; Black, Henry; Cushman, William; Green, Lee; Izzo Jr, Joseph; Jones, Daniel; Materson, Barry et al. "Seventh Report of the Joint National Committee on Prevention, Detection, Evaluation, and Treatment of High Blood Pressure." 42. (2003) Bethesda: U.S. Department of Health and Human Services. pp. 1206. doi:10.1161/01.HYP.0000107251.49515.c2. ISSN 0194-911X. PMID 14656957.

Eure, Marian Anne. "Making the DASH for Good Health," 2 April, 2010. http://seniorhealth.about.com/cs/nutrition/a/dash_diet.htm.

Heller, Marla. The DASH Diet Action Plan: Based on the National Institutes of Health Research, Dietary Approaches to Stop Hypertension. Deerfield, IL: Amidon Press, 2007. ISBN 978-0-9763408-1-2. OCLC 162507208.

Karanja, Njeri; Erlinger, TP; Pao-Hwa, Lin; Miller 3rd, Edgar R; Bray, George. "The DASH Diet for High Blood Pressure: From Clinical Trial to Dinner Table." Cleveland Clinic Journal of Medicine (Lyndhurst, Ohio: The Cleveland Clinic Foundation) 71 (2004): 745–53. DOI:10.3949/ccjm.71.9.745. ISSN 0891-1150. PMID 15478706.

Liebman, Bonnie. "DASH: A Diet for All Diseases." http://www.cspinet.org/nah/dash.htm.

Liese, Angela D., PhD, MPH; Nichols, Michele, MS; Sun, Xuezheng, MSPH' D'Agostino, Ralph B. Jr., PhD; Haffner, Steven M., MD. "Adherence to the DASH Diet Is Inversely Associated With Incidence of Type 2 Diabetes: The Insulin Resistance Atherosclerosis Study." American Diabetes Association, 1 June, 2009. http://care.diabetes journals.org/content/32/8/1434.full.

Medical News Today. "DASH Diet Comes Tops Overall, Followed by the Mediterranean Diet." 8 June, 2011. http://www.medicalnewstoday .com/articles/227945.php.

MedicineNet.com, "The DASH Diet." http://www.medicinenet.com/ the_dash_diet/article.htm.

Moore, Thomas; Svetkey, Laura; Appel, Lawrence; Bray, George; Volmer, William. The DASH Diet for Hypertension. New York: Simon & Schuster, 2001. ISBN 978-0-7432-0295-4. OCLC 47243951.

National Heart, Lung, and Blood Institute. "What Is the DASH Eating Plan?" 2 July, 2012. http://www.nhlbi.nih.gov/health/health-topics/ topics/dash/.

Nowlan, Sandra. Delicious DASH Flavours: The Proven, Drug-Free, Doctor-Recommended Approach to Reducing High Blood Pressure. Halifax N.S.: Formac, 2008. ISBN 978-0-88780-766-4. OCLC 185022611.

Pao-Hwa Lin*,3, Fiona Ginty†, Lawrence J. Appel**, Mikel Aickin‡, Arline Bohannon††, Patrick Garnero‡‡, Denis Barclay#, and Laura P. Svetkey*,"The DASH Diet and Sodium Reduction Improve Markers of Bone Turnover and Calcium Metabolism in Adults," Journal of Nutrition, 133 (2003): 3130–3136 http://jn.nutrition.org/ content/133/10/3130.full.

Pexton, Carolyn. "A Dash of This Diet Lowers Blood Pressure," 20 August, 2010. http://www.fyiliving.com/diet/a-dash-of-this-diet-lowers-blood-pressure/.

Reuters. "DASH Diet Best Overall in New Rankings." 7 June, 2011 http://www.reuters.com/article/2011/06/07/us-diets-report-idUSTRE75657C20110607.

Sacks, Frank M; Svetkey, Laura; Vollmer, William; Appel, Lawrence; Bray, George; Harsha, David; Obarzanek, Eva; Conlin, Paul et al. "Effects on Blood Pressure of Reduced Dietary Sodium and the Dietary Approaches to Stop Hypertension (DASH) Diet." New England Journal of Medicine (Massachusetts Medical Society sunshinehs) **344** (2001): 3–10. DOI:10.1056/NEJM200101043440101. ISSN 0028-4793. PMID 11136953.

Sacks, Frank M; Obarzanek, Eva; Windhauser, Marlene; Svetkey, Laura; Vollmer, William; McCullough, Marjorie; Karanja, Njeri; Lin, Pao-Hwa et al. "Rationale and Design of the Dietary Approaches to Stop Hypertension trial (DASH)." Annals of Epidemiology (Elsevier) **5** (1995): 108–118. DOI:10.1016/1047-2797(94)00055-X. ISSN 10472797. PMID 7795829.

United States Department of Health and Human Services. "Dietary Guidelines for Americans,"(PDF) 2005. http://www.health.gov/dietaryguidelines/dga2005/document/pdf/DGA2005.pdf.

University of Wisconsin School of Medicine and Public Health. "Which Diet Works: A Nutrition Review," 29 March, 2007. http://videos.med.wisc.edu/videos/195.

US Department of Health and Human Services. "Your Guide to Lowering Your Blood Pressure With DASH" (PDF), April 2006. http://www.nhlbi.nih.gov/health/public/heart/hbp/dash/new_dash.pdf.

US News Health. "DASH Diet." http://health.usnews.com/best-diet/ dash-diet.

Wikipedia. "DASH Diet." 8 May, 2012. http://en.wikipedia.org/wiki/ DASH_diet.

Women's Heart Foundation. "Dietary Approaches to Stop Hypertension." http://www.womensheart.org/content/Nutrition/dash_diet.asp.

Made in the USA
San Bernardino, CA
08 October 2017